ANXIETY DISORDERS

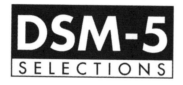

ANXIETY DISORDERS

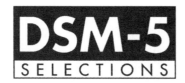

DSM-5
SELECTIONS

American Psychiatric Association

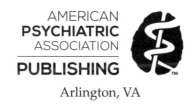

AMERICAN
PSYCHIATRIC
ASSOCIATION
PUBLISHING

Arlington, VA

Manufactured in the United States of America on acid-free paper.

ISBN 978-1-61537-014-6 (Paperback)

American Psychiatric Association
1000 Wilson Boulevard
Arlington, VA 22209-3901
www.psych.org

Anxiety Disorders: DSM-5® Selections is an anthology published by the American Psychiatric Association from the following sources:

American Psychiatric Association: *Diagnostic and Statistical Manual of Mental Disorders, Fifth Edition.* Arlington, VA, American Psychiatric Association, 2013

Black DW, Grant JE: *DSM-5® Guidebook: The Essential Companion to the Diagnostic and Statistical Manual of Mental Disorders, Fifth Edition.* Washington, DC, American Psychiatric Publishing, 2014

Barnhill JW: *DSM-5® Clinical Cases.* Washington, DC, American Psychiatric Publishing, 2014

Muskin PR: *DSM-5® Self-Exam Questions: Test Questions for the Diagnostic Criteria.* Washington, DC, American Psychiatric Publishing, 2014

Contents

Introduction to DSM-5® Selections

Welcome to *DSM-5 Selections*. The purpose of this series is to educate readers about important diagnostic issues associated with categories of DSM-5 disorders. The initial books in the *DSM-5 Selections* series are *Sleep-Wake Disorders, Depressive Disorders, Schizophrenia Spectrum and Other Psychotic Disorders, Feeding and Eating Disorders, Neurodevelopmental Disorders,* and *Anxiety Disorders.* Each book in the series includes the diagnostic criteria relevant to the disorders included in each category. The criteria are taken directly from DSM-5, the most comprehensive, current, and critical resource for clinical practice available today. Also included in each book in the series are extracts from the *DSM-5 Guidebook, DSM-5 Clinical Cases,* and *DSM-5 Self-Exam Questions.* Consequently, each book in the series offers readers a unique introduction to individual categories of DSM-5 disorders and an opportunity to test one's knowledge about DSM-5 disorders.

DSM-5 Guidebook serves as a roadmap to DSM-5 disorders for clinicians and researchers. It illuminates the content of DSM-5 by teaching mental health professionals how to use the revised diagnostic criteria, and it provides practical content for its clinical use. The book offers a fresh perspective to DSM diagnostic categories by focusing on the changes between DSM-IV-TR and DSM-5 that will most significantly impact clinical application of the criteria.

DSM-5 Clinical Cases presents composite patient cases that exemplify the diagnostic criteria for disorders contained in a category. *DSM-5 Clinical Cases* makes DSM-5 come alive for teachers, students, and clinicians. The book helps readers to understand diagnostic concepts, including symptoms, severity, comorbidities, age at onset and development, dimensionality across disorders, and gender and cultural implications.

The questions in *DSM-5 Self-Exam Questions* were written to test readers' knowledge of conceptual changes to DSM-5, specific changes to diagnoses, and the diagnostic criteria. Each question includes short answers that explain the rationale for each correct answer and contain important information on diagnostic classification, criteria sets, diagnoses, codes, severity, culture, age, and gender. The questions are helpful for preparing for various examinations.

The *DSM-5 Selections* series is not intended to replace DSM-5 or the other books from which the extracts are taken. Rather, the series is intended to give readers key selected materials that pertain directly to specific disorder categories. If you find that you require more information about a specific disorder or category of disorders, you are encouraged to examine an APP textbook or clinical manual. You can review the full list of APP titles at www.appi.org.

Robert E. Hales, M.D.
Editor-in-Chief

Preface

Anxiety disorders are an important and frequently occurring group of psychiatric disorders and are commonly encountered in clinical practice. In most studies of primary care settings, anxiety disorders (10%–15% of patients) are more common than depressive disorders (7%–10% of patients). Anxiety disorders are more frequent in women, with ratios of women to men between 1.4:1 and 1.8:1. The median age at onset of anxiety disorders is usually in the teens to 20s.

The most common anxiety disorders by lifetime prevalence are specific phobia (15.6%), followed by social anxiety disorder (social phobia) (10.7%), separation anxiety disorder (6.7%), generalized anxiety disorder (4.3%), panic disorder (3.8%), and agoraphobia (2.5%). Anxiety disorders associated with other conditions often lead to poorer outcomes.

In general psychiatry outpatient practice, anxiety disorders will comprise 40% of new referrals. Among the mental disorders, anxiety disorders are the most prevalent conditions in any age category. They are also associated with substantial cost to society due to disability and lost work productivity. Recent evidence shows that anxiety disorders are associated with an increased risk of suicidal behavior. Consequently, suicidality should always be assessed when evaluating a patient with an anxiety disorder.

Physical health conditions are common among patients with anxiety disorders. The most prevalent medical conditions are cardiovascular disease, respiratory illness, arthritis, and migraine headaches. In addition, the onset of serious physical illness may trigger the onset of an anxiety disorder.

The changes made to the DSM-5 diagnostic criteria for anxiety disorders are highlighted below. This is not meant to be an exhaustive guide to DSM-5 changes, and minor changes in text or wording made for clarity are not described. Section I of DSM-5 contains a full description of changes pertaining to the chapter organization in DSM-5, the multiaxial system, and the introduction of dimensional assessments.

Highlights of Changes From DSM-IV-TR to DSM-5

The DSM-5 chapter on anxiety disorders no longer includes obsessive-compulsive disorder (which is included with the obsessive-compulsive and related disorders) or posttraumatic stress disorder and acute stress disorder (which are included with the trauma- and stressor-related disorders). However, the sequential order of these chapters in DSM-5 reflects the close relationships among them.

Adapted with permission from Stein MB, Sareen J: "Anxiety Disorders," in *The American Psychiatric Publishing Textbook of Psychiatry*, 6th Edition. Edited by Hales RE, Yudofsky SC, Roberts LW. Washington, DC, American Psychiatric Publishing, 2014, pp. 391–429.

Agoraphobia, Specific Phobia, and Social Anxiety Disorder (Social Phobia)

Changes in criteria for agoraphobia, specific phobia, and social anxiety disorder (social phobia) include deletion of the requirement that individuals older than 18 years recognize that their anxiety is excessive or unreasonable. This change is based on evidence that individuals with such disorders often overestimate the danger in phobic situations and that older individuals often misattribute phobic fears to aging. Instead, the anxiety must be out of proportion to the actual danger or threat in the situation, after cultural contextual factors are taken into account. In addition, the 6-month duration, which was limited to individuals younger than 18 years in DSM-IV, is now extended to all ages. This change is intended to minimize overdiagnosis of transient fears.

Panic Attack

The essential features of panic attacks remain unchanged, although the complicated DSM-IV terminology for describing different types of panic attacks (i.e., situationally bound/cued, situationally predisposed, and unexpected/uncued) is replaced with the terms *unexpected* and *expected panic attacks.*

Panic attacks function as a marker and prognostic factor for severity of diagnosis, course, and comorbidity across an array of disorders, including but not limited to anxiety disorders. Hence, panic attack can be listed as a specifier that is applicable to all DSM-5 disorders.

Panic Disorder and Agoraphobia

Panic disorder and agoraphobia are unlinked in DSM-5. Thus, the former DSM-IV diagnoses of panic disorder with agoraphobia, panic disorder without agoraphobia, and agoraphobia without history of panic disorder are now replaced by two diagnoses, panic disorder and agoraphobia, each with separate criteria. The co-occurrence of panic disorder and agoraphobia is now coded with two diagnoses. This change recognizes that a substantial number of individuals with agoraphobia do not experience panic symptoms. The diagnostic criteria for agoraphobia are derived from the DSM-IV descriptors for agoraphobia, although endorsement of fears from two or more agoraphobia situations is now required because this is a robust means for distinguishing agoraphobia from specific phobia. Also, the criteria for agoraphobia are extended to be consistent with criteria sets for other anxiety disorders (e.g., clinician judgment of the fears as being out of proportion to the actual danger in the situation, with a typical duration of 6 months or more).

Specific Phobia

The core features of specific phobia remain the same, but there is no longer a requirement that individuals older than 18 years must recognize that their fear and anxiety are excessive or unreasonable, and the duration requirement ("typically lasting for 6 months or more") now applies to all ages. Although they are now referred to as specifiers, the different types of specific phobia have essentially remained unchanged.

Social Anxiety Disorder (Social Phobia)

The essential features of social anxiety disorder (social phobia) (formerly called *social phobia*) remain the same. However, a number of changes have been made, including deletion of the requirement that individuals older than 18 years must recognize that their fear or anxiety is excessive or unreasonable, and the duration criterion of "typically lasting for 6 months or more" is now required for all ages. A more significant change is that the *generalized* specifier has been deleted and replaced with a *performance only* specifier. The DSM-IV generalized specifier was problematic in that "fears include most social situations" was difficult to operationalize. Individuals who fear only performance situations (i.e., speaking or performing in front of an audience) appear to represent a distinct subset of social anxiety disorder in terms of etiology, age at onset, physiological response, and treatment response.

Separation Anxiety Disorder

Although in DSM-IV, separation anxiety disorder was classified in the section "Disorders Usually First Diagnosed in Infancy, Childhood, or Adolescence," it is now classified as an anxiety disorder. The core features remain mostly unchanged, although the wording of the criteria has been modified to more adequately represent the expression of separation anxiety symptoms in adulthood. For example, attachment figures may include the children of adults with separation anxiety disorder, and avoidance behaviors may occur in the workplace as well as at school. Also, in contrast to DSM-IV, in DSM-5 the diagnostic criteria no longer specify that age at onset must be before 18 years, because a substantial number of adults report onset of separation anxiety after age 18. Also, a duration criterion—"typically lasting for 6 months or more"—has been added for adults to minimize overdiagnosis of transient fears.

Selective Mutism

In DSM-IV, selective mutism was classified in the section "Disorders Usually First Diagnosed in Infancy, Childhood, or Adolescence." It is now classified as an anxiety disorder, given that a large majority of children with selective mutism are anxious. The diagnostic criteria are largely unchanged from DSM-IV.

DSM-5® Anxiety Disorders: ICD-9-CM and ICD-10-CM Codes

Disorder	ICD-9-CM	ICD-10-CM
Separation Anxiety Disorder	309.21	F93.0
Selective Mutism	313.23	F94.0
Specific Phobia		
Animal	300.29	F40.218
Natural environment	300.29	F40.228
Blood-injection-injury	300.29	F40.23x
Fear of blood		F40.230
Fear of injections and transfusions		F40.231
Fear of other medical care		F40.232
Fear of injury		F40.233
Situational	300.29	F40.248
Other	300.29	F40.298
Social Anxiety Disorder (Social Phobia)	300.23	F40.10
Panic Disorder	300.01	F41.0
Agoraphobia	300.22	F40.00
Generalized Anxiety Disorder	300.02	F41.1
Substance/Medication-Induced Anxiety Disorder	See table below	
Anxiety Disorder Due to Another Medical Condition	293.84	F06.4
Other Specified Anxiety Disorder	300.09	F41.8
Unspecified Anxiety Disorder	300.00	F41.9

Substance/Medication-Induced Anxiety Disorder

	ICD-9-CM	ICD-10-CM		
		With use disorder, mild	With use disorder, moderate or severe	Without use disorder
Alcohol	291.89	F10.180	F10.280	F10.980
Caffeine	292.89	F15.180	F15.280	F15.980
Cannabis	292.89	F12.180	F12.280	F12.980
Phencyclidine	292.89	F16.180	F16.280	F16.980
Other hallucinogen	292.89	F16.180	F16.280	F16.980
Inhalant	292.89	F18.180	F18.280	F18.980
Opioid	292.89	F11.188	F11.288	F11.988
Sedative, hypnotic, or anxiolytic	292.89	F13.180	F13.280	F13.980
Amphetamine (or other stimulant)	292.89	F15.180	F15.280	F15.980
Cocaine	292.89	F14.180	F14.280	F14.980
Other (or unknown) substance	292.89	F19.180	F19.280	F19.980

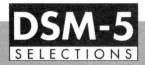

Anxiety Disorders
Diagnostic and Statistical Manual of Mental Disorders, Fifth Edition

Anxiety disorders include disorders that share features of excessive fear and anxiety and related behavioral disturbances. *Fear* is the emotional response to real or perceived imminent threat, whereas *anxiety* is anticipation of future threat. Obviously, these two states overlap, but they also differ, with fear more often associated with surges of autonomic arousal necessary for fight or flight, thoughts of immediate danger, and escape behaviors, and anxiety more often associated with muscle tension and vigilance in preparation for future danger and cautious or avoidant behaviors. Sometimes the level of fear or anxiety is reduced by pervasive avoidance behaviors. *Panic attacks* feature prominently within the anxiety disorders as a particular type of fear response. Panic attacks are not limited to anxiety disorders but rather can be seen in other mental disorders as well.

The anxiety disorders differ from one another in the types of objects or situations that induce fear, anxiety, or avoidance behavior, and the associated cognitive ideation. Thus, while the anxiety disorders tend to be highly comorbid with each other, they can be differentiated by close examination of the types of situations that are feared or avoided and the content of the associated thoughts or beliefs.

Anxiety disorders differ from developmentally normative fear or anxiety by being excessive or persisting beyond developmentally appropriate periods. They differ from transient fear or anxiety, often stress-induced, by being persistent (e.g., typically lasting 6 months or more), although the criterion for duration is intended as a general guide with allowance for some degree of flexibility and is sometimes of shorter duration in children (as in separation anxiety disorder and selective mutism). Since individuals with anxiety disorders typically overestimate the danger in situations they fear or avoid, the primary determination of whether the fear or anxiety is excessive or out of proportion is made by the clinician, taking cultural contextual factors into account. Many of the anxiety disorders develop in childhood and tend to persist if not treated. Most occur more frequently in females than in males (approximately 2:1 ratio). Each anxiety disorder is diagnosed only when the symptoms are not attributable to the physiological effects of a substance/medication or to another medical condition or are not better explained by another mental disorder.

The chapter is arranged developmentally, with disorders sequenced according to the typical age at onset. The individual with separation anxiety disorder is fearful or anxious about separation from attachment figures to a degree that is developmentally inappropriate. There is persistent fear or anxiety about harm coming to attachment figures and events that could lead to loss of or separation from attachment figures and reluctance to go away from attachment figures, as well as nightmares and physical symptoms of distress. Although the symptoms often develop in childhood, they can be expressed throughout adulthood as well.

Selective mutism is characterized by a consistent failure to speak in social situations in which there is an expectation to speak (e.g., school) even though the individual speaks in other situations. The failure to speak has significant consequences on achievement in academic or occupational settings or otherwise interferes with normal social communication.

Individuals with specific phobia are fearful or anxious about or avoidant of circumscribed objects or situations. A specific cognitive ideation is not featured in this disorder, as it is in other anxiety disorders. The fear, anxiety, or avoidance is almost always immediately induced by the phobic situation, to a degree that is persistent and out of proportion to the actual risk posed. There are various types of specific phobias: animal; natural environment; blood-injection-injury; situational; and other situations.

In social anxiety disorder (social phobia), the individual is fearful or anxious about or avoidant of social interactions and situations that involve the possibility of being scrutinized. These include social interactions such as meeting unfamiliar people, situations in which the individual may be observed eating or drinking, and situations in which the individual performs in front of others. The cognitive ideation is of being negatively evaluated by others, by being embarrassed, humiliated, or rejected, or offending others.

In panic disorder, the individual experiences recurrent unexpected panic attacks and is persistently concerned or worried about having more panic attacks or changes his or her behavior in maladaptive ways because of the panic attacks (e.g., avoidance of exercise or of unfamiliar locations). Panic attacks are abrupt surges of intense fear or intense discomfort that reach a peak within minutes, accompanied by physical and/or cognitive symptoms. Limited-symptom panic attacks include fewer than four symptoms. Panic attacks may be *expected,* such as in response to a typically feared object or situation, or *unexpected,* meaning that the panic attack occurs for no apparent reason. Panic attacks function as a marker and prognostic factor for severity of diagnosis, course, and comorbidity across an array of disorders, including, but not limited to, the anxiety disorders (e.g., substance use, depressive and psychotic disorders). Panic attack may therefore be used as a descriptive specifier for any anxiety disorder as well as other mental disorders.

Individuals with agoraphobia are fearful and anxious about two or more of the following situations: using public transportation; being in open spaces; being in enclosed places; standing in line or being in a crowd; or being outside of the home alone in other situations. The individual fears these situations because of thoughts that escape might be difficult or help might not be available in the event of developing panic-like symptoms or other incapacitating or embarrassing symptoms. These situations almost always induce fear or anxiety and are often avoided or require the presence of a companion.

The key features of generalized anxiety disorder are persistent and excessive anxiety and worry about various domains, including work and school performance, that the individual finds difficult to control. In addition, the individual experiences physical symptoms, including restlessness or feeling keyed up or on edge; being easily fatigued; difficulty concentrating or mind going blank; irritability; muscle tension; and sleep disturbance.

Substance/medication-induced anxiety disorder involves anxiety due to substance intoxication or withdrawal or to a medication treatment. In anxiety disorder due to another medical condition, anxiety symptoms are the physiological consequence of another medical condition.

Disorder-specific scales are available to better characterize the severity of each anxiety disorder and to capture change in severity over time. For ease of use, particularly for individuals with more than one anxiety disorder, these scales have been developed to have the same format (but different focus) across the anxiety disorders, with ratings of behavioral symptoms, cognitive ideation symptoms, and physical symptoms relevant to each disorder.

Separation Anxiety Disorder

Diagnostic Criteria   309.21 (F93.0)

A. Developmentally inappropriate and excessive fear or anxiety concerning separation from those to whom the individual is attached, as evidenced by at least three of the following:

1. Recurrent excessive distress when anticipating or experiencing separation from home or from major attachment figures.
2. Persistent and excessive worry about losing major attachment figures or about possible harm to them, such as illness, injury, disasters, or death.
3. Persistent and excessive worry about experiencing an untoward event (e.g., getting lost, being kidnapped, having an accident, becoming ill) that causes separation from a major attachment figure.
4. Persistent reluctance or refusal to go out, away from home, to school, to work, or elsewhere because of fear of separation.
5. Persistent and excessive fear of or reluctance about being alone or without major attachment figures at home or in other settings.
6. Persistent reluctance or refusal to sleep away from home or to go to sleep without being near a major attachment figure.
7. Repeated nightmares involving the theme of separation.
8. Repeated complaints of physical symptoms (e.g., headaches, stomachaches, nausea, vomiting) when separation from major attachment figures occurs or is anticipated.

B. The fear, anxiety, or avoidance is persistent, lasting at least 4 weeks in children and adolescents and typically 6 months or more in adults.

C. The disturbance causes clinically significant distress or impairment in social, academic, occupational, or other important areas of functioning.

D. The disturbance is not better explained by another mental disorder, such as refusing to leave home because of excessive resistance to change in autism spectrum disorder; delusions or hallucinations concerning separation in psychotic disorders; refusal to go outside without a trusted companion in agoraphobia; worries about ill health or other harm befalling significant others in generalized anxiety disorder; or concerns about having an illness in illness anxiety disorder.

Diagnostic Features

The essential feature of separation anxiety disorder is excessive fear or anxiety concerning separation from home or attachment figures. The anxiety exceeds what may be expected given the person's developmental level (Criterion A). Individuals with separation anxiety disorder have symptoms that meet at least three of the following criteria: They experience recurrent excessive distress when separation from home or major attachment figures is anticipated or occurs (Criterion A1). They worry about the well-being or death of attachment figures, particularly when separated from them, and they need to know the whereabouts of their attachment figures and want to stay in touch with them (Criterion A2). They also worry about untoward events to themselves, such as getting lost, being kidnapped, or having an accident, that would keep them from ever being reunited with their major attachment figure (Criterion A3). Individuals with separation anxiety disorder are reluctant or refuse to go out by themselves because of separation fears (Criterion A4). They have persistent and excessive fear or reluctance about being alone or without major attachment figures at home or in other settings. Children with separation anxiety disorder may be unable to stay or go in a room by themselves and may display "clinging" behavior, staying close to or "shadowing" the parent around the house, or requiring someone to be with them when going to another room in the house (Criterion A5). They have persistent reluctance or refusal to go to sleep without being near a major attachment figure or to sleep away from home (Criterion A6). Children with this disorder often have difficulty at bedtime and may insist that someone stay with them until they fall asleep. During the night, they may make their way to their parents' bed (or that of a significant other, such as a sibling). Children may be reluctant or refuse to attend camp, to sleep at friends' homes, or to go on errands. Adults may be uncomfortable when traveling independently (e.g., sleeping in a hotel room). There may be repeated nightmares in which the content expresses the individual's separation anxiety (e.g., destruction of the family through fire, murder, or other catastrophe) (Criterion A7). Physical symptoms (e.g., headaches, abdominal complaints, nausea, vomiting) are common in children when separation from major attachment figures occurs or is anticipated (Criterion A8). Cardiovascular symptoms such as palpitations, dizziness, and feeling faint are rare in younger children but may occur in adolescents and adults.

The disturbance must last for a period of at least 4 weeks in children and adolescents younger than 18 years and is typically 6 months or longer in adults (Criterion B). However, the duration criterion for adults should be used as a general guide, with allowance for some degree of flexibility. The disturbance must cause clinically significant distress or impairment in social, academic, occupational, or other important areas of functioning (Criterion C).

Associated Features Supporting Diagnosis

When separated from major attachment figures, children with separation anxiety disorder may exhibit social withdrawal, apathy, sadness, or difficulty concentrating on work or play. Depending on their age, individuals may have fears of animals, monsters, the dark, muggers, burglars, kidnappers, car accidents, plane travel, and other situations that are perceived as presenting danger to the family or themselves. Some individuals become homesick and uncomfortable to the point of misery when away from home. Separation anxiety disorder in children may lead to school refusal, which in turn may lead to academic difficulties and social isolation. When extremely upset at the prospect of separation, children may show anger or occasionally aggression toward someone who is forcing separation. When alone, especially in the evening or the dark, young children may report unusual perceptual experiences (e.g., seeing people peering into their room, frightening creatures reaching for them, feeling eyes staring at them). Children with this disorder may be described as demanding, intrusive, and in need of constant attention, and, as adults, may appear dependent and overprotective. The individual's excessive demands often become a source of frustration for family members, leading to resentment and conflict in the family.

Prevalence

The 12-month prevalence of separation anxiety disorder among adults in the United States is 0.9%–1.9%. In children, 6- to 12-month prevalence is estimated to be approximately 4%. In adolescents in the United States, the 12-month prevalence is 1.6%. Separation anxiety disorder decreases in prevalence from childhood through adolescence and adulthood and is the most prevalent anxiety disorder in children younger than 12 years. In clinical samples of children, the disorder is equally common in males and females. In the community, the disorder is more frequent in females.

Development and Course

Periods of heightened separation anxiety from attachment figures are part of normal early development and may indicate the development of secure attachment relationships (e.g., around 1 year of age, when infants may suffer from stranger anxiety). Onset of separation anxiety disorder may be as early as preschool age and may occur at any time during childhood and more rarely in adolescence. Typically there are periods of exacerbation and remission. In some cases, both the anxiety about possible separation and the avoidance of situations involving separation from the home or nuclear family (e.g., going away to college, moving away from attachment figures) may persist through adulthood. However, the majority of children with separation anxiety disorder are free of impairing anxiety disorders over their lifetimes. Many adults with separation anxiety disorder do not recall a childhood onset of separation anxiety disorder, although they may recall symptoms.

The manifestations of separation anxiety disorder vary with age. Younger children are more reluctant to go to school or may avoid school altogether. Younger children may not express worries or specific fears of definite threats to parents, home, or themselves, and the anxiety is manifested only when separation is experienced. As children age, worries emerge; these are often worries about specific dangers (e.g., accidents, kidnapping, mugging, death) or vague concerns about not being reunited with attachment figures. In adults, separation anxiety disorder may limit their ability to cope with changes in circumstances (e.g., moving, getting married). Adults with the disorder are typically overconcerned about their offspring and spouses and experience marked discomfort when separated from them. They may also experience significant disruption in work or social experiences because of needing to continuously check on the whereabouts of a significant other.

Risk and Prognostic Factors

Environmental.   Separation anxiety disorder often develops after life stress, especially a loss (e.g., the death of a relative or pet; an illness of the individual or a relative; a change of schools; parental divorce; a move to a new neighborhood; immigration; a disaster that involved periods of separation from attachment figures). In young adults, other examples of life stress include leaving the parental home, entering into a romantic relationship, and becoming a parent. Parental overprotection and intrusiveness may be associated with separation anxiety disorder.

Genetic and physiological.   Separation anxiety disorder in children may be heritable. Heritability was estimated at 73% in a community sample of 6-year-old twins, with higher rates in girls. Children with separation anxiety disorder display particularly enhanced sensitivity to respiratory stimulation using CO_2-enriched air.

Culture-Related Diagnostic Issues

There are cultural variations in the degree to which it is considered desirable to tolerate separation, so that demands and opportunities for separation between parents and children are avoided in some cultures. For example, there is wide variation across countries and cultures with respect to the age at which it is expected that offspring should leave the parental home. It is important to differentiate separation anxiety disorder from the high value some cultures place on strong interdependence among family members.

Gender-Related Diagnostic Issues

Girls manifest greater reluctance to attend or avoidance of school than boys. Indirect expression of fear of separation may be more common in males than in females, for example, by limited independent activity, reluctance to be away from home alone, or distress when spouse or offspring do things independently or when contact with spouse or offspring is not possible.

Suicide Risk

Separation anxiety disorder in children may be associated with an increased risk for suicide. In a community sample, the presence of mood disorders, anxiety disorders, or substance use has been associated with suicidal ideation and attempts. However, this association is not specific to separation anxiety disorder and is found in several anxiety disorders.

Functional Consequences of Separation Anxiety Disorder

Individuals with separation anxiety disorder often limit independent activities away from home or attachment figures (e.g., in children, avoiding school, not going to camp, having difficulty sleeping alone; in adolescents, not going away to college; in adults, not leaving the parental home, not traveling, not working outside the home).

Differential Diagnosis

Generalized anxiety disorder. Separation anxiety disorder is distinguished from generalized anxiety disorder in that the anxiety predominantly concerns separation from attachment figures, and if other worries occur, they do not predominate the clinical picture.

Panic disorder. Threats of separation may lead to extreme anxiety and even a panic attack. In separation anxiety disorder, in contrast to panic disorder, the anxiety concerns the possibility of being away from attachment figures and worry about untoward events befalling them, rather than being incapacitated by an unexpected panic attack.

Agoraphobia. Unlike individuals with agoraphobia, those with separation anxiety disorder are not anxious about being trapped or incapacitated in situations from which escape is perceived as difficult in the event of panic-like symptoms or other incapacitating symptoms.

Conduct disorder. School avoidance (truancy) is common in conduct disorder, but anxiety about separation is not responsible for school absences, and the child or adolescent usually stays away from, rather than returns to, the home.

Social anxiety disorder. School refusal may be due to social anxiety disorder (social phobia). In such instances, the school avoidance is due to fear of being judged negatively by others rather than to worries about being separated from the attachment figures.

Posttraumatic stress disorder. Fear of separation from loved ones is common after traumatic events such as a disasters, particularly when periods of separation from loved ones were experienced during the traumatic event. In PTSD, the central symptoms concern intrusions about, and avoidance of, memories associated with the traumatic event itself, whereas in separation anxiety disorder, the worries and avoidance concern the well-being of attachment figures and separation from them.

Illness anxiety disorder. Individuals with illness anxiety disorder worry about specific illnesses they may have, but the main concern is about the medical diagnosis itself, not about being separated from attachment figures.

Bereavement. Intense yearning or longing for the deceased, intense sorrow and emotional pain, and preoccupation with the deceased or the circumstances of the death are expected responses occurring in bereavement, whereas fear of separation from other attachment figures is central in separation anxiety disorder.

Depressive and bipolar disorders. These disorders may be associated with reluctance to leave home, but the main concern is not worry or fear of untoward events befalling attachment figures, but rather low motivation for engaging with the outside world. However, individuals with separation anxiety disorder may become depressed while being separated or in anticipation of separation.

Oppositional defiant disorder. Children and adolescents with separation anxiety disorder may be oppositional in the context of being forced to separate from attachment figures. Oppositional defiant disorder should be considered only when there is persistent oppositional behavior unrelated to the anticipation or occurrence of separation from attachment figures.

Psychotic disorders.   Unlike the hallucinations in psychotic disorders, the unusual perceptual experiences that may occur in separation anxiety disorder are usually based on a misperception of an actual stimulus, occur only in certain situations (e.g., nighttime), and are reversed by the presence of an attachment figure.

Personality disorders.   Dependent personality disorder is characterized by an indiscriminate tendency to rely on others, whereas separation anxiety disorder involves concern about the proximity and safety of main attachment figures. Borderline personality disorder is characterized by fear of abandonment by loved ones, but problems in identity, self-direction, interpersonal functioning, and impulsivity are additionally central to that disorder, whereas they are not central to separation anxiety disorder.

Comorbidity

In children, separation anxiety disorder is highly comorbid with generalized anxiety disorder and specific phobia. In adults, common comorbidities include specific phobia, PTSD, panic disorder, generalized anxiety disorder, social anxiety disorder, agoraphobia, obsessive-compulsive disorder, and personality disorders. Depressive and bipolar disorders are also comorbid with separation anxiety disorder in adults.

Selective Mutism

Diagnostic Criteria   **313.23** (F94.0)

A. Consistent failure to speak in specific social situations in which there is an expectation for speaking (e.g., at school) despite speaking in other situations.
B. The disturbance interferes with educational or occupational achievement or with social communication.
C. The duration of the disturbance is at least 1 month (not limited to the first month of school).
D. The failure to speak is not attributable to a lack of knowledge of, or comfort with, the spoken language required in the social situation.
E. The disturbance is not better explained by a communication disorder (e.g., childhood-onset fluency disorder) and does not occur exclusively during the course of autism spectrum disorder, schizophrenia, or another psychotic disorder.

Diagnostic Features

When encountering other individuals in social interactions, children with selective mutism do not initiate speech or reciprocally respond when spoken to by others. Lack of speech occurs in social interactions with children or adults. Children with selective mutism will speak in their home in the presence of immediate family members but often not even in front of close friends or second-degree relatives, such as grandparents or cousins. The disturbance is often marked by high social anxiety. Children with selective mutism often refuse to speak at school, leading to academic or educational impairment, as teachers often find it difficult to assess skills such as reading. The lack of speech may interfere with social communication, although children with this disorder sometimes use nonspoken or nonverbal means (e.g., grunting, pointing, writing) to communicate and may be willing or eager to perform or engage in social encounters when speech is not required (e.g., nonverbal parts in school plays).

Associated Features Supporting Diagnosis

Associated features of selective mutism may include excessive shyness, fear of social embarrassment, social isolation and withdrawal, clinging, compulsive traits, negativism, temper tantrums, or mild oppositional behavior. Although children with this disorder generally have normal language skills, there may occasionally be an associated communication disorder, although no particular association with a specific communication disorder has been identified. Even when these disorders are present, anxiety is present as well. In clinical settings, children with selective mutism are almost always given an additional diagnosis of another anxiety disorder—most commonly, social anxiety disorder (social phobia).

Prevalence

Selective mutism is a relatively rare disorder and has not been included as a diagnostic category in epidemiological studies of prevalence of childhood disorders. Point prevalence using various clinic or school samples ranges between 0.03% and 1% depending on the setting (e.g., clinic vs. school vs. general population) and ages of the individuals in the sample. The prevalence of the disorder does not seem to vary by sex or race/ethnicity. The disorder is more likely to manifest in young children than in adolescents and adults.

Development and Course

The onset of selective mutism is usually before age 5 years, but the disturbance may not come to clinical attention until entry into school, where there is an increase in social interaction and performance tasks, such as reading aloud. The persistence of the disorder is variable. Although clinical reports suggest that many individuals "outgrow" selective mutism, the longitudinal course of the disorder is unknown. In some cases, particularly in individuals with social anxiety disorder, selective mutism may disappear, but symptoms of social anxiety disorder remain.

Risk and Prognostic Factors

Temperamental. Temperamental risk factors for selective mutism are not well identified. Negative affectivity (neuroticism) or behavioral inhibition may play a role, as may parental history of shyness, social isolation, and social anxiety. Children with selective mutism may have subtle receptive language difficulties compared with their peers, although receptive language is still within the normal range.

Environmental. Social inhibition on the part of parents may serve as a model for social reticence and selective mutism in children. Furthermore, parents of children with selective mutism have been described as overprotective or more controlling than parents of children with other anxiety disorders or no disorder.

Genetic and physiological factors.   Because of the significant overlap between selective mutism and social anxiety disorder, there may be shared genetic factors between these conditions.

Culture-Related Diagnostic Issues

Children in families who have immigrated to a country where a different language is
spoken may refuse to speak the new language because of lack of knowledge of the language. If comprehension of the new language is adequate but refusal to speak persists, a diagnosis of selective mutism may be warranted.

Functional Consequences of Selective Mutism

Selective mutism may result in social impairment, as children may be too anxious to
engage in reciprocal social interaction with other children. As children with selective
mutism mature, they may face increasing social isolation. In school settings, these
children may suffer academic impairment, because often they do not communicate
with teachers regarding their academic or personal needs (e.g., not understanding a
class assignment, not asking to use the restroom). Severe impairment in school and social functioning, including that resulting from teasing by peers, is common. In certain
instances, selective mutism may serve as a compensatory strategy to decrease anxious
arousal in social encounters.

Differential Diagnosis

Communication disorders.   Selective mutism should be distinguished from speech
disturbances that are better explained by a communication disorder, such as language
disorder, speech sound disorder (previously phonological disorder), childhood-onset
fluency disorder (stuttering), or pragmatic (social) communication disorder. Unlike
selective mutism, the speech disturbance in these conditions is not restricted to a specific social situation.

Neurodevelopmental disorders and schizophrenia and other psychotic disorders.
Individuals with an autism spectrum disorder, schizophrenia or another psychotic disorder, or severe intellectual disability may have problems in social communication and
be unable to speak appropriately in social situations. In contrast, selective mutism
should be diagnosed only when a child has an established capacity to speak in some social situations (e.g., typically at home).

Social anxiety disorder (social phobia).   The social anxiety and social avoidance in
social anxiety disorder may be associated with selective mutism. In such cases, both
diagnoses may be given.

Comorbidity

The most common comorbid conditions are other anxiety disorders, most commonly
social anxiety disorder, followed by separation anxiety disorder and specific phobia.
Oppositional behaviors have been noted to occur in children with selective mutism, although oppositional behavior may be limited to situations requiring speech. Communication delays or disorders also may appear in some children with selective mutism.

Specific Phobia

Diagnostic Criteria

A. Marked fear or anxiety about a specific object or situation (e.g., flying, heights, animals, receiving an injection, seeing blood).

Note: In children, the fear or anxiety may be expressed by crying, tantrums, freezing, or clinging.

B. The phobic object or situation almost always provokes immediate fear or anxiety.

C. The phobic object or situation is actively avoided or endured with intense fear or anxiety.

D. The fear or anxiety is out of proportion to the actual danger posed by the specific object or situation and to the sociocultural context.

E. The fear, anxiety, or avoidance is persistent, typically lasting for 6 months or more.

F. The fear, anxiety, or avoidance causes clinically significant distress or impairment in social, occupational, or other important areas of functioning.

G. The disturbance is not better explained by the symptoms of another mental disorder, including fear, anxiety, and avoidance of situations associated with panic-like symptoms or other incapacitating symptoms (as in agoraphobia); objects or situations related to obsessions (as in obsessive-compulsive disorder); reminders of traumatic events (as in posttraumatic stress disorder); separation from home or attachment figures (as in separation anxiety disorder); or social situations (as in social anxiety disorder).

Specify if:
Code based on the phobic stimulus:

300.29 (F40.218) Animal (e.g., spiders, insects, dogs).

300.29 (F40.228) Natural environment (e.g., heights, storms, water).

300.29 (F40.23x) Blood-injection-injury (e.g., needles, invasive medical procedures).

> **Coding note:** Select specific ICD-10-CM code as follows: **F40.230** fear of blood; **F40.231** fear of injections and transfusions; **F40.232** fear of other medical care; or **F40.233** fear of injury.

300.29 (F40.248) Situational (e.g., airplanes, elevators, enclosed places).

300.29 (F40.298) Other (e.g., situations that may lead to choking or vomiting; in children, e.g., loud sounds or costumed characters).

Coding note: When more than one phobic stimulus is present, code all ICD-10-CM codes that apply (e.g., for fear of snakes and flying, F40.218 specific phobia, animal, and F40.248 specific phobia, situational).

Specifiers

It is common for individuals to have multiple specific phobias. The average individual with specific phobia fears three objects or situations, and approximately 75% of individuals with specific phobia fear more than one situation or object. In such cases, multiple specific phobia diagnoses, each with its own diagnostic code reflecting the phobic stimulus, would need to be given. For example, if an individual fears thunderstorms and flying, then two diagnoses would be given: specific phobia, natural environment, and specific phobia, situational.

Diagnostic Features

A key feature of this disorder is that the fear or anxiety is circumscribed to the presence of a particular situation or object (Criterion A), which may be termed the *phobic stimulus.* The categories of feared situations or objects are provided as specifiers. Many individuals fear objects or situations from more than one category, or phobic stimulus. For the diagnosis of specific phobia, the response must differ from normal, transient fears that commonly occur in the population. To meet the criteria for a diagnosis, the fear or anxiety must be intense or severe (i.e., "marked") (Criterion A). The amount of fear experienced may vary with proximity to the feared object or situation and may occur in anticipation of or in the actual presence of the object or situation. Also, the fear or anxiety may take the form of a full or limited symptom panic attack (i.e., expected panic attack). Another characteristic of specific phobias is that fear or anxiety is evoked nearly every time the individual comes into contact with the phobic stimulus (Criterion B). Thus, an individual who becomes anxious only occasionally upon being confronted with the situation or object (e.g., becomes anxious when flying only on one out of every five airplane flights) would not be diagnosed with specific phobia. However, the degree of fear or anxiety expressed may vary (from anticipatory anxiety to a full panic attack) across different occasions of encountering the phobic object or situation because of various contextual factors such as the presence of others, duration of exposure, and other threatening elements such as turbulence on a flight for individuals who fear flying. Fear and anxiety are often expressed differently between children and adults. Also, the fear or anxiety occurs as soon as the phobic object or situation is encountered (i.e., immediately rather than being delayed).

The individual actively avoids the situation, or if he or she either is unable or decides not to avoid it, the situation or object evokes intense fear or anxiety (Criterion C). *Active avoidance* means the individual intentionally behaves in ways that are designed to prevent or minimize contact with phobic objects or situations (e.g., takes tunnels instead of bridges on daily commute to work for fear of heights; avoids entering a dark room for fear of spiders; avoids accepting a job in a locale where a phobic stimulus is more common). Avoidance behaviors are often obvious (e.g., an individual who fears blood refusing to go to the doctor) but are sometimes less obvious (e.g., an individual who fears snakes refusing to look at pictures that resemble the form or shape of snakes). Many individuals with specific phobias have suffered over many years and have changed their living circumstances in ways designed to avoid the phobic object or situation as much as possible (e.g., an individual diagnosed with specific phobia, animal, who moves to reside in an area devoid of the particular feared animal). Therefore, they no longer experience fear or anxiety in their daily life. In such instances, avoidance behaviors or ongoing refusal to engage in activities that would involve exposure to the phobic object or situation (e.g., repeated refusal to accept offers for work-related travel because of fear of flying) may be helpful in confirming the diagnosis in the absence of overt anxiety or panic.

The fear or anxiety is out of proportion to the actual danger that the object or situation poses, or more intense than is deemed necessary (Criterion D). Although individuals with specific phobia often recognize their reactions as disproportionate, they tend to overestimate the danger in their feared situations, and thus the judgment of being out of proportion is made by the clinician. The individual's sociocultural context should also be taken into account. For example, fears of the dark may be reasonable in a context of ongoing violence, and fear of insects may be more disproportionate in settings where insects are consumed in the diet. The fear, anxiety, or avoidance is persistent, typically lasting for 6 months or more (Criterion E), which helps distinguish the disorder from transient fears that are common in the population, particularly among children. However, the duration criterion should be used as a general guide, with allowance for some degree of flexibility. The specific phobia must cause clinically significant distress or impairment in social, occupational, or other important areas of functioning in order for the disorder to be diagnosed (Criterion F).

Associated Features Supporting Diagnosis

Individuals with specific phobia typically experience an increase in physiological arousal in anticipation of or during exposure to a phobic object or situation. However, the physiological response to the feared situation or object varies. Whereas individuals with situational, natural environment, and animal specific phobias are likely to show sympathetic nervous system arousal, individuals with blood-injection-injury specific phobia often demonstrate a vasovagal fainting or near-fainting response that is marked by initial brief acceleration of heart rate and elevation of blood pressure followed by a deceleration of heart rate and a drop in blood pressure. Current neural systems models for specific phobia emphasize the amygdala and related structures, much as in other anxiety disorders.

Prevalence

In the United States, the 12-month community prevalence estimate for specific phobia is approximately 7%–9%. Prevalence rates in European countries are largely similar to those in the United States (e.g., about 6%), but rates are generally lower in Asian, African, and Latin American countries (2%–4%). Prevalence rates are approximately 5% in children and are approximately 16% in 13- to 17-year-olds. Prevalence rates are lower in older individuals (about 3%–5%), possibly reflecting diminishing severity to subclinical levels. Females are more frequently affected than males, at a rate of approximately 2:1, although rates vary across different phobic stimuli. That is, animal, natural environment, and situational specific phobias are predominantly experienced by females, whereas blood-injection-injury phobia is experienced nearly equally by both genders.

Development and Course

Specific phobia sometimes develops following a traumatic event (e.g., being attacked by an animal or stuck in an elevator), observation of others going through a traumatic event (e.g., watching someone drown), an unexpected panic attack in the to be feared situation (e.g., an unexpected panic attack while on the subway), or informational transmission (e.g., extensive media coverage of a plane crash). However, many individuals with specific phobia are unable to recall the specific reason for the onset of their phobias. Specific phobia usually develops in early childhood, with the majority of cases developing prior to age 10 years. The median age at onset is between 7 and 11 years, with the mean at about 10 years. Situational specific phobias tend to have a later age at onset than natural environment, animal, or blood-injection-injury specific phobias. Specific phobias that develop in childhood and adolescence are likely to wax and wane during that period. However, phobias that do persist into adulthood are unlikely to remit for the majority of individuals.

When specific phobia is being diagnosed in children, two issues should be considered. First, young children may express their fear and anxiety by crying, tantrums, freezing, or clinging. Second, young children typically are not able to understand the concept of avoidance. Therefore, the clinician should assemble additional information from parents, teachers, or others who know the child well. Excessive fears are quite common in young children but are usually transitory and only mildly impairing and thus considered developmentally appropriate. In such cases a diagnosis of specific phobia would not be made. When the diagnosis of specific phobia is being considered in a child, it is important to assess the degree of impairment and the duration of the fear, anxiety, or avoidance, and whether it is typical for the child's particular developmental stage.

Although the prevalence of specific phobia is lower in older populations, it remains one of the more commonly experienced disorders in late life. Several issues should be considered when diagnosing specific phobia in older populations. First, older individuals may be more likely to endorse natural environment specific phobias, as well as phobias of falling. Second, specific phobia (like all anxiety disorders) tends to co-occur with medical concerns in older individuals, including coronary heart disease and chronic obstructive pulmonary disease. Third, older individuals may be more likely to attribute the symptoms of anxiety to medical conditions. Fourth, older individuals may be more likely to manifest anxiety in an atypical manner (e.g., involving symptoms of both anxiety and depression) and thus be more likely to warrant a diagnosis of unspecified anxiety disorder. Additionally, the presence of specific phobia in older adults is associated with decreased quality of life and may serve as a risk factor for major neurocognitive disorder.

Although most specific phobias develop in childhood and adolescence, it is possible for a specific phobia to develop at any age, often as the result of experiences that are traumatic. For example, phobias of choking almost always follow a near-choking event at any age.

Risk and Prognostic Factors

Temperamental. Temperamental risk factors for specific phobia, such as negative affectivity (neuroticism) or behavioral inhibition, are risk factors for other anxiety disorders as well.

Environmental. Environmental risk factors for specific phobias, such as parental overprotectiveness, parental loss and separation, and physical and sexual abuse, tend to predict other anxiety disorders as well. As noted earlier, negative or traumatic encounters with the feared object or situation sometimes (but not always) precede the development of specific phobia.

Genetic and physiological.   There may be a genetic susceptibility to a certain category of specific phobia (e.g., an individual with a first-degree relative with a specific phobia of animals is significantly more likely to have the same specific phobia than any other category of phobia). Individuals with blood-injection-injury phobia show a unique propensity to vasovagal syncope (fainting) in the presence of the phobic stimulus.

Culture-Related Diagnostic Issues

In the United States, Asians and Latinos report significantly lower rates of specific phobia than non-Latino whites, African Americans, and Native Americans. In addition to having lower prevalence rates of specific phobia, some countries outside of the United States, particularly Asian and African countries, show differing phobia content, age at onset, and gender ratios.

Suicide Risk

Individuals with specific phobia are up to 60% more likely to make a suicide attempt than are individuals without the diagnosis. However, it is likely that these elevated rates are primarily due to comorbidity with personality disorders and other anxiety disorders.

Functional Consequences of Specific Phobia

Individuals with specific phobia show similar patterns of impairment in psychosocial functioning and decreased quality of life as individuals with other anxiety disorders and alcohol and substance use disorders, including impairments in occupational and interpersonal functioning. In older adults, impairment may be seen in caregiving duties and volunteer activities. Also, fear of falling in older adults can lead to reduced mobility and reduced physical and social functioning, and may lead to receiving formal or informal home support. The distress and impairment caused by specific phobias tend to increase with the number of feared objects and situations. Thus, an individual who fears four objects or situations is likely to have more impairment in his or her occupational and social roles and a lower quality of life than an individual who fears only one object or situation. Individuals with blood-injection-injury specific phobia are often reluctant to obtain medical care even when a medical concern is present. Additionally, fear of vomiting and choking may substantially reduce dietary intake.

Differential Diagnosis

Agoraphobia.   Situational specific phobia may resemble agoraphobia in its clinical presentation, given the overlap in feared situations (e.g., flying, enclosed places, elevators). If an individual fears only one of the agoraphobia situations, then specific phobia, situational, may be diagnosed. If two or more agoraphobic situations are feared, a diagnosis of agoraphobia is likely warranted. For example, an individual who fears airplanes and elevators (which overlap with the "public transportation" agoraphobic situation) but does not fear other agoraphobic situations would be diagnosed with specific phobia, situational, whereas an individual who fears airplanes, elevators, and crowds (which overlap with two agoraphobic situations, "using public transportation" and "standing in line and or being in a crowd") would be diagnosed with agoraphobia. Criterion B of agoraphobia (the situations are feared or avoided "because of thoughts that escape might be difficult or help might not be available in the event of developing panic-like symptoms or other incapacitating or embarrassing symptoms") can also be useful in differentiating agoraphobia from specific phobia. If the situations are feared for other reasons, such as fear of being harmed directly by the object or situations (e.g., fear of the plane crashing, fear of the animal biting), a specific phobia diagnosis may be more appropriate.

Social anxiety disorder.   If the situations are feared because of negative evaluation, social anxiety disorder should be diagnosed instead of specific phobia.

Separation anxiety disorder.   If the situations are feared because of separation from a primary caregiver or attachment figure, separation anxiety disorder should be diagnosed instead of specific phobia.

Panic disorder.   Individuals with specific phobia may experience panic attacks when confronted with their feared situation or object. A diagnosis of specific phobia would be given if the panic attacks only occurred in response to the specific object or situation, whereas a diagnosis of panic disorder would be given if the individual also experienced panic attacks that were unexpected (i.e., not in response to the specific phobia object or situation).

Obsessive-compulsive disorder.   If an individual's primary fear or anxiety is of an object or situation as a result of obsessions (e.g., fear of blood due to obsessive thoughts about contamination from blood-borne pathogens [i.e., HIV]; fear of driving due to obsessive images of harming others), and if other diagnostic criteria for obsessive-compulsive disorder are met, then obsessive-compulsive disorder should be diagnosed.

Trauma- and stressor-related disorders.   If the phobia develops following a traumatic event, PTSD should be considered as a diagnosis. However, traumatic events can precede the onset of PTSD and specific phobia. In this case, a diagnosis of specific phobia would be assigned only if all of the criteria for PTSD are not met.

Eating disorders.   A diagnosis of specific phobia is not given if the avoidance behavior is exclusively limited to avoidance of food and food-related cues, in which case a diagnosis of anorexia nervosa or bulimia nervosa should be considered.

Schizophrenia spectrum and other psychotic disorders.   When the fear and avoidance are due to delusional thinking (as in schizophrenia or other schizophrenia spectrum and other psychotic disorders), a diagnosis of specific phobia is not warranted.

Comorbidity

Specific phobia is rarely seen in medical-clinical settings in the absence of other psychopathology and is more frequently seen in nonmedical mental health settings. Specific phobia is frequently associated with a range of other disorders, especially depression in older adults. Because of early onset, specific phobia is typically the temporally primary disorder. Individuals with specific phobia are at increased risk for the development of other disorders, including other anxiety disorders, depressive and bipolar disorders, substance-related disorders, somatic symptom and related disorders, and personality disorders (particularly dependent personality disorder).

Social Anxiety Disorder (Social Phobia)

Diagnostic Criteria   **300.23 (F40.10)**

A. Marked fear or anxiety about one or more social situations in which the individual is exposed to possible scrutiny by others. Examples include social interactions (e.g., having a conversation, meeting unfamiliar people), being observed (e.g., eating or drinking), and performing in front of others (e.g., giving a speech).

   Note: In children, the anxiety must occur in peer settings and not just during interactions with adults.

B. The individual fears that he or she will act in a way or show anxiety symptoms that will be negatively evaluated (i.e., will be humiliating or embarrassing; will lead to rejection or offend others).

C. The social situations almost always provoke fear or anxiety.

   Note: In children, the fear or anxiety may be expressed by crying, tantrums, freezing, clinging, shrinking, or failing to speak in social situations.

D. The social situations are avoided or endured with intense fear or anxiety.

E. The fear or anxiety is out of proportion to the actual threat posed by the social situation and to the sociocultural context.

F. The fear, anxiety, or avoidance is persistent, typically lasting for 6 months or more.

G. The fear, anxiety, or avoidance causes clinically significant distress or impairment in social, occupational, or other important areas of functioning.

H. The fear, anxiety, or avoidance is not attributable to the physiological effects of a substance (e.g., a drug of abuse, a medication) or another medical condition.

I. The fear, anxiety, or avoidance is not better explained by the symptoms of another mental disorder, such as panic disorder, body dysmorphic disorder, or autism spectrum disorder.

J. If another medical condition (e.g., Parkinson's disease, obesity, disfigurement from burns or injury) is present, the fear, anxiety, or avoidance is clearly unrelated or is excessive.

Specify if:

   Performance only: If the fear is restricted to speaking or performing in public.

Specifiers

Individuals with the performance only type of social anxiety disorder have performance fears that are typically most impairing in their professional lives (e.g., musicians, dancers, performers, athletes) or in roles that require regular public speaking. Performance fears may also manifest in work, school, or academic settings in which regular public presentations are required. Individuals with performance only social anxiety disorder do not fear or avoid nonperformance social situations.

Diagnostic Features

The essential feature of social anxiety disorder is a marked, or intense, fear or anxiety of social situations in which the individual may be scrutinized by others. In children the fear or anxiety must occur in peer settings and not just during interactions with adults (Criterion A). When exposed to such social situations, the individual fears that he or she will be negatively evaluated. The individual is concerned that he or she will be judged as anxious, weak, crazy, stupid, boring, intimidating, dirty, or unlikable. The individual fears that he or she will act or appear in a certain way or show anxiety symptoms, such as blushing, trembling, sweating, stumbling over one's words, or staring, that will be negatively evaluated by others (Criterion B). Some individuals fear offending others or being rejected as a result. Fear of offending others—for example, by a gaze or by showing anxiety symptoms—may be the predominant fear in individuals from cultures with strong collectivistic orientations. An individual with fear of trembling of the hands may avoid drinking, eating, writing, or pointing in public; an individual with fear of sweating may avoid shaking hands or eating spicy foods; and an individual with fear of blushing may avoid public performance, bright lights, or discussion about intimate topics. Some individuals fear and avoid urinating in public restrooms when other individuals are present (i.e., paruresis, or "shy bladder syndrome").

The social situations almost always provoke fear or anxiety (Criterion C). Thus, an individual who becomes anxious only occasionally in the social situation(s) would not be diagnosed with social anxiety disorder. However, the degree and type of fear and anxiety may vary (e.g., anticipatory anxiety, a panic attack) across different occasions. The anticipatory anxiety may occur sometimes far in advance of upcoming situations (e.g., worrying every day for weeks before attending a social event, repeating a speech for days in advance). In children, the fear or anxiety may be expressed by crying, tantrums, freezing, clinging, or shrinking in social situations. The individual will often avoid the feared social situations. Alternatively, the situations are endured with intense fear or anxiety (Criterion D). Avoidance can be extensive (e.g., not going to parties, refusing school) or subtle (e.g., overpreparing the text of a speech, diverting attention to others, limiting eye contact).

The fear or anxiety is judged to be out of proportion to the actual risk of being negatively evaluated or to the consequences of such negative evaluation (Criterion E). Sometimes, the anxiety may not be judged to be excessive, because it is related to an actual danger (e.g., being bullied or tormented by others). However, individuals with social anxiety disorder often overestimate the negative consequences of social situations, and thus the judgment of being out of proportion is made by the clinician. The individual's sociocultural context needs to be taken into account when this judgment is being made. For example, in certain cultures, behavior that might otherwise appear socially anxious may be considered appropriate in social situations (e.g., might be seen as a sign of respect).

The duration of the disturbance is typically at least 6 months (Criterion F). This duration threshold helps distinguish the disorder from transient social fears that are common, particularly among children and in the community. However, the duration criterion should be used as a general guide, with allowance for some degree of flexibility. The fear, anxiety, and avoidance must interfere significantly with the individual's normal routine, occupational or academic functioning, or social activities or relationships, or must cause clinically significant distress or impairment in social, occupational, or other important areas of functioning (Criterion G). For example, an individual who is afraid to speak in public would not receive a diagnosis of social anxiety disorder if this activity is not routinely encountered on the job or in classroom work, and if the individual is not significantly distressed about it. However, if the individual avoids, or is passed over for, the job or education he or she really wants because of social anxiety symptoms, Criterion G is met.

Associated Features Supporting Diagnosis

Individuals with social anxiety disorder may be inadequately assertive or excessively submissive or, less commonly, highly controlling of the conversation. They may show overly rigid body posture or inadequate eye contact, or speak with an overly soft voice. These individuals may be shy or withdrawn, and they may be less open in conversations and disclose little about themselves. They may seek employment in jobs that do not require social contact, although this is not the case for individuals with social anxiety disorder, performance only. They may live at home longer. Men may be delayed in marrying and having a family, whereas women who would want to work outside the home may live a life as homemaker and mother. Self-medication with substances is common (e.g., drinking before going to a party). Social anxiety among older adults may also include exacerbation of symptoms of medical illnesses, such as increased tremor or tachycardia. Blushing is a hallmark physical response of social anxiety disorder.

Prevalence

The 12-month prevalence estimate of social anxiety disorder for the United States is approximately 7%. Lower 12-month prevalence estimates are seen in much of the world using the same diagnostic instrument, clustering around 0.5%–2.0%; median prevalence in Europe is 2.3%. The 12-month prevalence rates in children and adolescents are comparable to those in adults. Prevalence rates decrease with age. The 12-month prevalence for older adults ranges from 2% to 5%. In general, higher rates of social anxiety disorder are found in females than in males in the general population (with odds ratios ranging from 1.5 to 2.2), and the gender difference in prevalence is more pronounced in adolescents and young adults. Gender rates are equivalent or slightly higher for males in clinical samples, and it is assumed that gender roles and social expectations play a significant role in explaining the heightened help-seeking behavior in male patients. Prevalence in the United States is higher in American Indians and lower in persons of Asian, Latino, African American, and Afro-Caribbean descent compared with non-Hispanic whites.

Development and Course

Median age at onset of social anxiety disorder in the United States is 13 years, and 75% of individuals have an age at onset between 8 and 15 years. The disorder sometimes emerges out of a childhood history of social inhibition or shyness in U.S. and European studies. Onset can also occur in early childhood. Onset of social anxiety disorder may follow a stressful or humiliating experience (e.g., being bullied, vomiting during a public speech), or it may be insidious, developing slowly. First onset in adulthood is relatively rare and is more likely to occur after a stressful or humiliating event or after life changes that require new social roles (e.g., marrying someone from a different social class, receiving a job promotion). Social anxiety disorder may diminish after an individual with fear of dating marries and may reemerge after divorce. Among individuals presenting to clinical care, the disorder tends to be particularly persistent.

Adolescents endorse a broader pattern of fear and avoidance, including of dating, compared with younger children. Older adults express social anxiety at lower levels but across a broader range of situations, whereas younger adults express higher levels of social anxiety for specific situations. In older adults, social anxiety may concern disability due to declining sensory functioning (hearing, vision) or embarrassment about one's appearance (e.g., tremor as a symptom of Parkinson's disease) or functioning due to medical conditions, incontinence, or cognitive impairment (e.g., forgetting people's names). In the community approximately 30% of individuals with social anxiety disorder experience remission of symptoms within 1 year, and about 50% experience remission within a few years. For approximately 60% of individuals without a specific treatment for social anxiety disorder, the course takes several years or longer.

Detection of social anxiety disorder in older adults may be challenging because of several factors, including a focus on somatic symptoms, comorbid medical illness, limited insight, changes to social environment or roles that may obscure impairment in social functioning, or reticence about describing psychological distress.

Risk and Prognostic Factors

Temperamental.   Underlying traits that predispose individuals to social anxiety disorder include behavioral inhibition and fear of negative evaluation.

Environmental.   There is no causative role of increased rates of childhood maltreatment or other early-onset psychosocial adversity in the development of social anxiety disorder. However, childhood maltreatment and adversity are risk factors for social anxiety disorder.

Genetic and physiological.   Traits predisposing individuals to social anxiety disorder, such as behavioral inhibition, are strongly genetically influenced. The genetic influence is subject to gene-environment interaction; that is, children with high behavioral inhibition are more susceptible to environmental influences, such as socially anxious modeling by parents. Also, social anxiety disorder is heritable (but performance-only anxiety less so). First-degree relatives have a two to six times greater chance of having social anxiety disorder, and liability to the disorder involves the interplay of disorder-specific (e.g., fear of negative evaluation) and nonspecific (e.g., neuroticism) genetic factors.

Culture-Related Diagnostic Issues

The syndrome of *taijin kyofusho* (e.g., in Japan and Korea) is often characterized by social-evaluative concerns, fulfilling criteria for social anxiety disorder, that are associated with the fear that the individual makes *other* people uncomfortable (e.g., "My gaze upsets people so they look away and avoid me"), a fear that is at times experienced with delusional intensity. This symptom may also be found in non-Asian settings. Other presentations of *taijin kyofusho* may fulfill criteria for body dysmorphic disorder or delusional disorder. Immigrant status is associated with significantly lower rates of social anxiety disorder in both Latino and non-Latino white groups. Prevalence rates of social anxiety disorder may not be in line with self-reported social anxiety levels in the same culture—that is, societies with strong collectivistic orientations may report high levels of social anxiety but low prevalence of social anxiety disorder.

Gender-Related Diagnostic Issues

Females with social anxiety disorder report a greater number of social fears and co-morbid depressive, bipolar, and anxiety disorders, whereas males are more likely to fear dating, have oppositional defiant disorder or conduct disorder, and use alcohol and illicit drugs to relieve symptoms of the disorder. Paruresis is more common in males.

Functional Consequences of Social Anxiety Disorder

Social anxiety disorder is associated with elevated rates of school dropout and with decreased well-being, employment, workplace productivity, socioeconomic status, and quality of life. Social anxiety disorder is also associated with being single, unmarried, or divorced and with not having children, particularly among men. In older adults, there may be impairment in caregiving duties and volunteer activities. Social anxiety disorder also impedes leisure activities. Despite the extent of distress and social impairment associated with social anxiety disorder, only about half of individuals with the disorder in Western societies ever seek treatment, and they tend to do so only after 15–20 years of experiencing symptoms. Not being employed is a strong predictor for the persistence of social anxiety disorder.

Differential Diagnosis

Normative shyness. Shyness (i.e., social reticence) is a common personality trait and is not by itself pathological. In some societies, shyness is even evaluated positively. However, when there is a significant adverse impact on social, occupational, and other important areas of functioning, a diagnosis of social anxiety disorder should be considered, and when full diagnostic criteria for social anxiety disorder are met, the disorder should be diagnosed. Only a minority (12%) of self-identified shy individuals in the United States have symptoms that meet diagnostic criteria for social anxiety disorder.

Agoraphobia. Individuals with agoraphobia may fear and avoid social situations (e.g., going to a movie) because escape might be difficult or help might not be available in the event of incapacitation or panic-like symptoms, whereas individuals with social anxiety disorder are most fearful of scrutiny by others. Moreover, individuals with social anxiety disorder are likely to be calm when left entirely alone, which is often not the case in agoraphobia.

Panic disorder.   Individuals with social anxiety disorder may have panic attacks, but the concern is about fear of negative evaluation, whereas in panic disorder the concern is about the panic attacks themselves.

Generalized anxiety disorder.   Social worries are common in generalized anxiety disorder, but the focus is more on the nature of ongoing relationships rather than on fear of negative evaluation. Individuals with generalized anxiety disorder, particularly children, may have excessive worries about the quality of their social performance, but these worries also pertain to nonsocial performance and when the individual is not being evaluated by others. In social anxiety disorder, the worries focus on social performance and others' evaluation.

Separation anxiety disorder.   Individuals with separation anxiety disorder may avoid social settings (including school refusal) because of concerns about being separated from attachment figures or, in children, about requiring the presence of a parent when it is not developmentally appropriate. Individuals with separation anxiety disorder are usually comfortable in social settings when their attachment figure is present or when they are at home, whereas those with social anxiety disorder may be uncomfortable when social situations occur at home or in the presence of attachment figures.

Specific phobias.   Individuals with specific phobias may fear embarrassment or humiliation (e.g., embarrassment about fainting when they have their blood drawn), but they do not generally fear negative evaluation in other social situations.

Selective mutism.   Individuals with selective mutism may fail to speak because of fear of negative evaluation, but they do not fear negative evaluation in social situations where no speaking is required (e.g., nonverbal play).

Major depressive disorder.   Individuals with major depressive disorder may be concerned about being negatively evaluated by others because they feel they are bad or not worthy of being liked. In contrast, individuals with social anxiety disorder are worried about being negatively evaluated because of certain social behaviors or physical symptoms.

Body dysmorphic disorder.   Individuals with body dysmorphic disorder are preoccupied with one or more perceived defects or flaws in their physical appearance that are not observable or appear slight to others; this preoccupation often causes social anxiety and avoidance. If their social fears and avoidance are caused only by their beliefs about their appearance, a separate diagnosis of social anxiety disorder is not warranted.

Delusional disorder.   Individuals with delusional disorder may have nonbizarre delusions and/or hallucinations related to the delusional theme that focus on being rejected by or offending others. Although extent of insight into beliefs about social situations may vary, many individuals with social anxiety disorder have good insight that their beliefs are out of proportion to the actual threat posed by the social situation.

Autism spectrum disorder.   Social anxiety and social communication deficits are hallmarks of autism spectrum disorder. Individuals with social anxiety disorder typically have adequate age-appropriate social relationships and social communication capacity, although they may appear to have impairment in these areas when first interacting with unfamiliar peers or adults.

Personality disorders.   Given its frequent onset in childhood and its persistence into and through adulthood, social anxiety disorder may resemble a personality disorder. The most apparent overlap is with avoidant personality disorder. Individuals with avoidant personality disorder have a broader avoidance pattern than those with social anxiety disorder. Nonetheless, social anxiety disorder is typically more comorbid with avoidant personality disorder than with other personality disorders, and avoidant personality disorder is more comorbid with social anxiety disorder than with other anxiety disorders.

Other mental disorders.   Social fears and discomfort can occur as part of schizophrenia, but other evidence for psychotic symptoms is usually present. In individuals with an eating disorder, it is important to determine that fear of negative evaluation about eating disorder symptoms or behaviors (e.g., purging and vomiting) is not the sole source of social anxiety before applying a diagnosis of social anxiety disorder. Similarly, obsessive-compulsive disorder may be associated with social anxiety, but the additional diagnosis of social anxiety disorder is used only when social fears and avoidance are independent of the foci of the obsessions and compulsions.

Other medical conditions.   Medical conditions may produce symptoms that may be embarrassing (e.g. trembling in Parkinson's disease). When the fear of negative evaluation due to other medical conditions is excessive, a diagnosis of social anxiety disorder should be considered.

Oppositional defiant disorder.   Refusal to speak due to opposition to authority figures should be differentiated from failure to speak due to fear of negative evaluation.

Comorbidity

Social anxiety disorder is often comorbid with other anxiety disorders, major depressive disorder, and substance use disorders, and the onset of social anxiety disorder generally precedes that of the other disorders, except for specific phobia and separation anxiety disorder. Chronic social isolation in the course of a social anxiety disorder may result in major depressive disorder. Comorbidity with depression is high also in older adults. Substances may be used as self-medication for social fears, but the symptoms of substance intoxication or withdrawal, such as trembling, may also be a source of (further) social fear. Social anxiety disorder is frequently comorbid with bipolar disorder or body dysmorphic disorder; for example, an individual has body dysmorphic disorder concerning a preoccupation with a slight irregularity of her nose, as well as social anxiety disorder because of a severe fear of sounding unintelligent. The more generalized form of social anxiety disorder, but not social anxiety disorder, performance only, is often comorbid with avoidant personality disorder. In children, comorbidities with high-functioning autism and selective mutism are common.

Panic Disorder

Diagnostic Criteria   **300.01** (F41.0)

A. Recurrent unexpected panic attacks. A panic attack is an abrupt surge of intense fear or intense discomfort that reaches a peak within minutes, and during which time four (or more) of the following symptoms occur:

Note: The abrupt surge can occur from a calm state or an anxious state.

1. Palpitations, pounding heart, or accelerated heart rate.
2. Sweating.
3. Trembling or shaking.
4. Sensations of shortness of breath or smothering.
5. Feelings of choking.
6. Chest pain or discomfort.
7. Nausea or abdominal distress.
8. Feeling dizzy, unsteady, light-headed, or faint.
9. Chills or heat sensations.
10. Paresthesias (numbness or tingling sensations).
11. Derealization (feelings of unreality) or depersonalization (being detached from oneself).
12. Fear of losing control or "going crazy."
13. Fear of dying.

Note: Culture-specific symptoms (e.g., tinnitus, neck soreness, headache, uncontrollable screaming or crying) may be seen. Such symptoms should not count as one of the four required symptoms.

B. At least one of the attacks has been followed by 1 month (or more) of one or both of the following:

1. Persistent concern or worry about additional panic attacks or their consequences (e.g., losing control, having a heart attack, "going crazy").
2. A significant maladaptive change in behavior related to the attacks (e.g., behaviors designed to avoid having panic attacks, such as avoidance of exercise or unfamiliar situations).

C. The disturbance is not attributable to the physiological effects of a substance (e.g., a drug of abuse, a medication) or another medical condition (e.g., hyperthyroidism, cardiopulmonary disorders).

D. The disturbance is not better explained by another mental disorder (e.g., the panic attacks do not occur only in response to feared social situations, as in social anxiety disorder; in response to circumscribed phobic objects or situations, as in specific phobia; in response to obsessions, as in obsessive-compulsive disorder; in response to reminders of traumatic events, as in posttraumatic stress disorder; or in response to separation from attachment figures, as in separation anxiety disorder).

Diagnostic Features

Panic disorder refers to recurrent unexpected panic attacks (Criterion A). A panic attack is an abrupt surge of intense fear or intense discomfort that reaches a peak within minutes, and during which time four or more of a list of 13 physical and cognitive symptoms occur. The term *recurrent* literally means more than one unexpected panic attack. The term *unexpected* refers to a panic attack for which there is no obvious cue or trigger at the time of occurrence—that is, the attack appears to occur from out of the blue, such as when the individual is relaxing or emerging from sleep (nocturnal panic attack). In contrast, *expected* panic attacks are attacks for which there is an obvious cue or trigger, such as a situation in which panic attacks typically occur. The determination of whether panic attacks are expected or unexpected is made by the clinician, who makes this judgment based on a combination of careful questioning as to the sequence of events preceding or leading up to the attack and the individual's own judgment of whether or not the attack seemed to occur for no apparent reason. Cultural interpretations may influence the assignment of panic attacks as expected or unexpected (see section "Culture-Related Diagnostic Issues" for this disorder). In the United States and Europe, approximately one-half of individuals with panic disorder have expected panic attacks as well as unexpected panic attacks. Thus, the presence of expected panic attacks does not rule out the diagnosis of panic disorder. For more details regarding expected versus unexpected panic attacks, see the text accompanying panic attacks.

The frequency and severity of panic attacks vary widely. In terms of frequency, there may be moderately frequent attacks (e.g., one per week) for months at a time, or short bursts of more frequent attacks (e.g., daily) separated by weeks or months without any attacks or with less frequent attacks (e.g., two per month) over many years. Persons who have infrequent panic attacks resemble persons with more frequent panic attacks in terms of panic attack symptoms, demographic characteristics, comorbidity with other disorders, family history, and biological data. In terms of severity, individuals with panic disorder may have both full-symptom (four or more symptoms) and limited-symptom (fewer than four symptoms) attacks, and the number and type of panic attack symptoms frequently differ from one panic attack to the next. However, more than one unexpected full-symptom panic attack is required for the diagnosis of panic disorder.

The worries about panic attacks or their consequences usually pertain to physical concerns, such as worry that panic attacks reflect the presence of life-threatening illnesses (e.g., cardiac disease, seizure disorder); social concerns, such as embarrassment or fear of being judged negatively by others because of visible panic symptoms; and concerns about mental functioning, such as "going crazy" or losing control (Criterion B). The maladaptive changes in behavior represent attempts to minimize or avoid panic attacks or their consequences. Examples include avoiding physical exertion, reorganizing daily life to ensure that help is available in the event of a panic attack, restricting usual daily activities, and avoiding agoraphobia-type situations, such as leaving home, using public transportation, or shopping. If agoraphobia is present, a separate diagnosis of agoraphobia is given.

Associated Features Supporting Diagnosis

One type of unexpected panic attack is a *nocturnal* panic attack (i.e., waking from sleep in a state of panic, which differs from panicking after fully waking from sleep). In the United States, this type of panic attack has been estimated to occur at least one time in roughly one-quarter to one-third of individuals with panic disorder, of whom the majority also have daytime panic attacks. In addition to worry about panic attacks and their consequences, many individuals with panic disorder report constant or intermittent feelings of anxiety that are more broadly related to health and mental health concerns. For example, individuals with panic disorder often anticipate a catastrophic outcome from a mild physical symptom or medication side effect (e.g., thinking that they may have heart disease or that a headache means presence of a brain tumor). Such individuals often are relatively intolerant of medication side effects. In addition, there may be pervasive concerns about abilities to complete daily tasks or withstand daily stressors, excessive use of drugs (e.g., alcohol, prescribed medications or illicit drugs) to control panic attacks, or extreme behaviors aimed at controlling panic attacks (e.g., severe restrictions on food intake or avoidance of specific foods or medications because of concerns about physical symptoms that provoke panic attacks).

Prevalence

In the general population, the 12-month prevalence estimate for panic disorder across the United States and several European countries is about 2%–3% in adults and adolescents. In the United States, significantly lower rates of panic disorder are reported among Latinos, African Americans, Caribbean blacks, and Asian Americans, compared with non-Latino whites; American Indians, by contrast, have significantly higher rates. Lower estimates have been reported for Asian, African, and Latin American countries, ranging from 0.1% to 0.8%. Females are more frequently affected than males, at a rate of approximately 2:1. The gender differentiation occurs in adolescence and is already observable before age 14 years. Although panic attacks occur in children, the overall prevalence of panic disorder is low before age 14 years (<0.4%). The rates of panic disorder show a gradual increase during adolescence, particularly in females, and possibly following the onset of puberty, and peak during adulthood. The prevalence rates decline in older individuals (i.e., 0.7% in adults over the age of 64), possibly reflecting diminishing severity to subclinical levels.

Development and Course

The median age at onset for panic disorder in the United States is 20–24 years. A small number of cases begin in childhood, and onset after age 45 years is unusual but can occur. The usual course, if the disorder is untreated, is chronic but waxing and waning. Some individuals may have episodic outbreaks with years of remission in between, and others may have continuous severe symptomatology. Only a minority of individuals have full remission without subsequent relapse within a few years. The course of panic disorder typically is complicated by a range of other disorders, in particular other anxiety disorders, depressive disorders, and substance use disorders (see section "Comorbidity" for this disorder).

   Although panic disorder is very rare in childhood, first occurrence of "fearful spells" is often dated retrospectively back to childhood. As in adults, panic disorder in adolescents tends to have a chronic course and is frequently comorbid with other anxiety, depressive, and bipolar disorders. To date, no differences in the clinical presentation between adolescents and adults have been found. However, adolescents may be less worried about additional panic attacks than are young adults. Lower prevalence of panic disorder in older adults appears to be attributable to age-related "dampening" of the autonomic nervous system response. Many older individuals with "panicky feelings" are observed to have a "hybrid" of limited-symptom panic attacks and generalized anxiety. Also, older adults tend to attribute their panic attacks to certain stressful situations, such as a medical procedure or social setting. Older individuals may retrospectively endorse explanations for the panic attack (which would preclude the diagnosis of panic disorder), even if an attack might actually have been unexpected in the moment (and thus qualify as the basis for a panic disorder diagnosis). This may result in under-endorsement of unexpected panic attacks in older individuals. Thus, careful questioning of older adults is required to assess whether panic attacks were expected before entering the situation, so that unexpected panic attacks and the diagnosis of panic disorder are not overlooked.

While the low rate of panic disorder in children could relate to difficulties in symptom reporting, this seems unlikely given that children are capable of reporting intense fear or panic in relation to separation and to phobic objects or phobic situations. Adolescents might be less willing than adults to openly discuss panic attacks. Therefore, clinicians should be aware that unexpected panic attacks do occur in adolescents, much as they do in adults, and be attuned to this possibility when encountering adolescents presenting with episodes of intense fear or distress.

Risk and Prognostic Factors

Temperamental.   Negative affectivity (neuroticism) (i.e., proneness to experiencing negative emotions) and anxiety sensitivity (i.e., the disposition to believe that symptoms of anxiety are harmful) are risk factors for the onset of panic attacks and, separately, for worry about panic, although their risk status for the diagnosis of panic disorder is unknown. History of "fearful spells" (i.e., limited-symptom attacks that do not meet full criteria for a panic attack) may be a risk factor for later panic attacks and panic disorder. Although separation anxiety in childhood, especially when severe, may precede the later development of panic disorder, it is not a consistent risk factor.

Environmental.   Reports of childhood experiences of sexual and physical abuse are more common in panic disorder than in certain other anxiety disorders. Smoking is a risk factor for panic attacks and panic disorder. Most individuals report identifiable stressors in the months before their first panic attack (e.g., interpersonal stressors and stressors related to physical well-being, such as negative experiences with illicit or prescription drugs, disease, or death in the family).

Genetic and physiological.   It is believed that multiple genes confer vulnerability to panic disorder. However, the exact genes, gene products, or functions related to the genetic regions implicated remain unknown. Current neural systems models for panic disorder emphasize the amygdala and related structures, much as in other anxiety disorders. There is an increased risk for panic disorder among offspring of parents with anxiety, depressive, and bipolar disorders. Respiratory disturbance, such as asthma, is associated with panic disorder, in terms of past history, comorbidity, and family history.

Culture-Related Diagnostic Issues

The rate of fears about mental and somatic symptoms of anxiety appears to vary across cultures and may influence the rate of panic attacks and panic disorder. Also, cultural expectations may influence the classification of panic attacks as expected or unexpected. For example, a Vietnamese individual who has a panic attack after walking out into a windy environment (*trúng gió;* "hit by the wind") may attribute the panic attack to exposure to wind as a result of the cultural syndrome that links these two experiences, resulting in classification of the panic attack as expected. Various other cultural syndromes are associated with panic disorder, including *ataque de nervios* ("attack of nerves") among Latin Americans and *khyâl* attacks and "soul loss" among Cambodians. *Ataque de nervios* may involve trembling, uncontrollable screaming or crying, aggressive or suicidal behavior, and depersonalization or derealization, which may be experienced longer than the few minutes typical of panic attacks. Some clinical presentations of *ataque de nervios* fulfill criteria for conditions other than panic attack (e.g., other specified dissociative disorder). These syndromes impact the symptoms and frequency of panic disorder, including the individual's attribution of unexpectedness, as cultural syndromes may create fear of certain situations, ranging from interpersonal arguments (associated with *ataque de nervios*), to types of exertion (associated with *khyâl* attacks), to atmospheric wind (associated with *trúng gió* attacks). Clarification of the details of cultural attributions may aid in distinguishing expected and unexpected panic attacks. For more information regarding cultural syndromes, refer to the "Glossary of Cultural Concepts of Distress" in the Appendix [in DSM-5].

The specific worries about panic attacks or their consequences are likely to vary from one culture to another (and across different age groups and gender). For panic disorder, U.S. community samples of non-Latino whites have significantly less functional impairment than African Americans. There are also higher rates of objectively defined severity in non-Latino Caribbean blacks with panic disorder, and lower rates of panic disorder overall in both African American and Afro-Caribbean groups, suggesting that among individuals of African descent, the criteria for panic disorder may be met only when there is substantial severity and impairment.

Gender-Related Diagnostic Issues

The clinical features of panic disorder do not appear to differ between males and females. There is some evidence for sexual dimorphism, with an association between panic disorder and the catechol-O-methyltransferase (COMT) gene in females only.

Diagnostic Markers

Agents with disparate mechanisms of action, such as sodium lactate, caffeine, isoproterenol, yohimbine, carbon dioxide, and cholecystokinin, provoke panic attacks in individuals with panic disorder to a much greater extent than in healthy control subjects (and in some cases, than in individuals with other anxiety, depressive, or bipolar disorders without panic attacks). Also, for a proportion of individuals with panic disorder, panic attacks are related to hypersensitive medullary carbon dioxide detectors, resulting in hypocapnia and other respiratory irregularities. However, none of these laboratory findings are considered diagnostic of panic disorder.

Suicide Risk

Panic attacks and a diagnosis of panic disorder in the past 12 months are related to a higher rate of suicide attempts and suicidal ideation in the past 12 months even when comorbidity and a history of childhood abuse and other suicide risk factors are taken into account.

Functional Consequences of Panic Disorder

Panic disorder is associated with high levels of social, occupational, and physical disability; considerable economic costs; and the highest number of medical visits among the anxiety disorders, although the effects are strongest with the presence of agoraphobia. Individuals with panic disorder may be frequently absent from work or school for doctor and emergency room visits, which can lead to unemployment or dropping out of school. In older adults, impairment may be seen in caregiving duties or volunteer activities. Full-symptom panic attacks typically are associated with greater morbidity (e.g., greater health care utilization, more disability, poorer quality of life) than limited-symptom attacks.

Differential Diagnosis

Other specified anxiety disorder or unspecified anxiety disorder. Panic disorder should not be diagnosed if full-symptom (unexpected) panic attacks have never been experienced. In the case of only limited-symptom unexpected panic attacks, an other specified anxiety disorder or unspecified anxiety disorder diagnosis should be considered.

Anxiety disorder due to another medical condition. Panic disorder is not diagnosed if the panic attacks are judged to be a direct physiological consequence of another medical condition. Examples of medical conditions that can cause panic attacks include hyperthyroidism, hyperparathyroidism, pheochromocytoma, vestibular dysfunctions, seizure disorders, and cardiopulmonary conditions (e.g., arrhythmias, supraventricular tachycardia, asthma, chronic obstructive pulmonary disease [COPD]). Appropriate laboratory tests (e.g., serum calcium levels for hyperparathyroidism; Holter monitor for arrhythmias) or physical examinations (e.g., for cardiac conditions) may be helpful in determining the etiological role of another medical condition.

Substance/medication-induced anxiety disorder. Panic disorder is not diagnosed if the panic attacks are judged to be a direct physiological consequence of a substance. Intoxication with central nervous system stimulants (e.g., cocaine, amphetamines, caffeine) or cannabis and withdrawal from central nervous system depressants (e.g., alcohol, barbiturates) can precipitate a panic attack. However, if panic attacks continue to occur outside of the context of substance use (e.g., long after the effects of intoxication or withdrawal have ended), a diagnosis of panic disorder should be considered. In addition, because panic disorder may precede substance use in some individuals and may be associated with increased substance use, especially for purposes of self-medication, a detailed history should be taken to determine if the individual had panic attacks prior to excessive substance use. If this is the case, a diagnosis of panic disorder should be considered in addition to a diagnosis of substance use disorder. Features such as onset after age 45 years or the presence of atypical symptoms during a panic attack (e.g., vertigo, loss of consciousness, loss of bladder or bowel control, slurred speech, amnesia) suggest the possibility that another medical condition or a substance may be causing the panic attack symptoms.

Other mental disorders with panic attacks as an associated feature (e.g., other anxiety disorders and psychotic disorders).   Panic attacks that occur as a symptom of other anxiety disorders are expected (e.g., triggered by social situations in social anxiety disorder, by phobic objects or situations in specific phobia or agoraphobia, by worry in generalized anxiety disorder, by separation from home or attachment figures in separation anxiety disorder) and thus would not meet criteria for panic disorder. (**Note:** Sometimes an unexpected panic attack is associated with the onset of another anxiety disorder, but then the attacks become expected, whereas panic disorder is characterized by recurrent unexpected panic attacks.) If the panic attacks occur only in response to specific triggers, then only the relevant anxiety disorder is assigned. However, if the individual experiences unexpected panic attacks as well and shows persistent concern and worry or behavioral change because of the attacks, then an additional diagnosis of panic disorder should be considered.

Comorbidity

Panic disorder infrequently occurs in clinical settings in the absence of other psychopathology. The prevalence of panic disorder is elevated in individuals with other disorders, particularly other anxiety disorders (and especially agoraphobia), major depression, bipolar disorder, and possibly mild alcohol use disorder. While panic disorder often has an earlier age at onset than the comorbid disorder(s), onset sometimes occurs after the comorbid disorder and may be seen as a severity marker of the comorbid illness.

Reported lifetime rates of comorbidity between major depressive disorder and panic disorder vary widely, ranging from 10% to 65% in individuals with panic disorder. In approximately one-third of individuals with both disorders, the depression precedes the onset of panic disorder. In the remaining two-thirds, depression occurs coincident with or following the onset of panic disorder. A subset of individuals with panic disorder develop a substance-related disorder, which for some represents an attempt to treat their anxiety with alcohol or medications. Comorbidity with other anxiety disorders and illness anxiety disorder is also common.

Panic disorder is significantly comorbid with numerous general medical symptoms and conditions, including, but not limited to, dizziness, cardiac arrhythmias, hyperthyroidism, asthma, COPD, and irritable bowel syndrome. However, the nature of the association (e.g., cause and effect) between panic disorder and these conditions remains unclear. Although mitral valve prolapse and thyroid disease are more common among individuals with panic disorder than in the general population, the differences in prevalence are not consistent.

Panic Attack Specifier

Note: Symptoms are presented for the purpose of identifying a panic attack; however, panic attack is not a mental disorder and cannot be coded. Panic attacks can occur in the context of any anxiety disorder as well as other mental disorders (e.g., depressive disorders, posttraumatic stress disorder, substance use disorders) and some medical conditions (e.g., cardiac, respiratory, vestibular, gastrointestinal). When the presence of a panic attack is identified, it should be noted as a specifier (e.g., "posttraumatic stress disorder with panic attacks"). For panic disorder, the presence of panic attack is contained within the criteria for the disorder and panic attack is not used as a specifier.

An abrupt surge of intense fear or intense discomfort that reaches a peak within minutes, and during which time four (or more) of the following symptoms occur:

Note: The abrupt surge can occur from a calm state or an anxious state.

1. Palpitations, pounding heart, or accelerated heart rate.
2. Sweating.
3. Trembling or shaking.
4. Sensations of shortness of breath or smothering.
5. Feelings of choking.
6. Chest pain or discomfort.
7. Nausea or abdominal distress.
8. Feeling dizzy, unsteady, light-headed, or faint.
9. Chills or heat sensations.
10. Paresthesias (numbness or tingling sensations).
11. Derealization (feelings of unreality) or depersonalization (being detached from oneself).
12. Fear of losing control or "going crazy."
13. Fear of dying.

Note: Culture-specific symptoms (e.g., tinnitus, neck soreness, headache, uncontrollable screaming or crying) may be seen. Such symptoms should not count as one of the four required symptoms.

Features

The essential feature of a panic attack is an abrupt surge of intense fear or intense discomfort that reaches a peak within minutes and during which time four or more of 13 physical and cognitive symptoms occur. Eleven of these 13 symptoms are physical (e.g., palpitations, sweating), while two are cognitive (i.e., fear of losing control or going crazy, fear of dying). "Fear of going crazy" is a colloquialism often used by individuals with panic attacks and is not intended as a pejorative or diagnostic term. The term *within minutes* means that the time to peak intensity is literally only a few minutes. A panic attack can arise from either a calm state or an anxious state, and time to peak intensity should be assessed independently of any preceding anxiety. That is, the start of the panic attack is the point at which there is an abrupt increase in discomfort rather than the point at which anxiety first developed. Likewise, a panic attack can return to either an anxious state or a calm state and possibly peak again. A panic attack is distinguished from ongoing anxiety by its time to peak intensity, which occurs within minutes; its discrete nature; and its typically greater severity. Attacks that meet all other criteria but have fewer than four physical and/or cognitive symptoms are referred to as *limited-symptom attacks*.

There are two characteristic types of panic attacks: expected and unexpected. *Expected panic attacks* are attacks for which there is an obvious cue or trigger, such as situations in which panic attacks have typically occurred. *Unexpected panic attacks* are those for which there is no obvious cue or trigger at the time of occurrence (e.g., when relaxing or out of sleep [nocturnal panic attack]). The determination of whether panic attacks are expected or unexpected is made by the clinician, who makes this judgment based on a combination of careful questioning as to the sequence of events preceding or leading up to the attack and the individual's own judgment of whether or not the attack seemed to occur for no apparent reason. Cultural interpretations may influence their determination as expected or unexpected. Culture-specific symptoms (e.g., tinnitus, neck soreness, headache, uncontrollable screaming or crying) may be seen; however, such symptoms should not count as one of the four required symptoms. Panic attacks can occur in the context of any mental disorder (e.g., anxiety disorders, depressive disorders, bipolar disorders, eating disorders, obsessive-compulsive and related disorders, personality disorders, psychotic disorders, substance use disorders) and some medical conditions (e.g., cardiac, respiratory, vestibular, gastrointestinal), with the majority never meeting criteria for panic disorder. Recurrent unexpected panic attacks are required for a diagnosis of panic disorder.

Associated Features

One type of unexpected panic attack is a *nocturnal panic attack* (i.e., waking from sleep in a state of panic), which differs from panicking after fully waking from sleep. Panic attacks are related to a higher rate of suicide attempts and suicidal ideation even when comorbidity and other suicide risk factors are taken into account.

Prevalence

In the general population, 12-month prevalence estimates for panic attacks in the United States is 11.2% in adults. Twelve-month prevalence estimates do not appear to differ significantly among African Americans, Asian Americans, and Latinos. Lower 12-month prevalence estimates for European countries appear to range from 2.7% to 3.3%. Females are more frequently affected than males, although this gender difference is more pronounced for panic disorder. Panic attacks can occur in children but are relatively rare until the age of puberty, when the prevalence rates increase. The prevalence rates decline in older individuals, possibly reflecting diminishing severity to subclinical levels.

Development and Course

The mean age at onset for panic attacks in the United States is approximately 22–23 years among adults. However, the course of panic attacks is likely influenced by the course of any co-occurring mental disorder(s) and stressful life events. Panic attacks are uncommon, and unexpected panic attacks are rare, in preadolescent children. Adolescents might be less willing than adults to openly discuss panic attacks, even though they present with episodes of intense fear or discomfort. Lower prevalence of panic attacks in older individuals may be related to a weaker autonomic response to emotional states relative to younger individuals. Older individuals may be less inclined to use the word "fear" and more inclined to use the word "discomfort" to describe panic attacks. Older individuals with "panicky feelings" may have a hybrid of limited-symptom attacks and generalized anxiety. In addition, older individuals tend to attribute panic attacks to certain situations that are stressful (e.g., medical procedures, social settings) and may retrospectively endorse explanations for the panic attack even if it was unexpected in the moment. This may result in under-endorsement of unexpected panic attacks in older individuals.

Risk and Prognostic Factors

Temperamental.   Negative affectivity (neuroticism) (i.e., proneness to experiencing negative emotions) and anxiety sensitivity (i.e., the disposition to believe that symptoms of anxiety are harmful) are risk factors for the onset of panic attacks. History of "fearful spells" (i.e., limited-symptom attacks that do not meet full criteria for a panic attack) may be a risk factor for later panic attacks.

Environmental.   Smoking is a risk factor for panic attacks. Most individuals report identifiable stressors in the months before their first panic attack (e.g., interpersonal stressors and stressors related to physical well-being, such as negative experiences with illicit or prescription drugs, disease, or death in the family).

Culture-Related Diagnostic Issues

Cultural interpretations may influence the determination of panic attacks as expected or unexpected. Culture-specific symptoms (e.g., tinnitus, neck soreness, headache, and uncontrollable screaming or crying) may be seen; however, such symptoms should not count as one of the four required symptoms. Frequency of each of the 13 symptoms varies cross-culturally (e.g., higher rates of paresthesias in African Americans and of dizziness in several Asian groups). Cultural syndromes also influence the cross-cultural presentation of panic attacks, resulting in different symptom profiles across different cultural groups. Examples include *khyâl* (wind) attacks, a Cambodian cultural syndrome involving dizziness, tinnitus, and neck soreness; and *trúng gió* (wind-related) attacks, a Vietnamese cultural syndrome associated with headaches. *Ataque de nervios* (attack of nerves) is a cultural syndrome among Latin Americans that may involve trembling, uncontrollable screaming or crying, aggressive or suicidal behavior, and depersonalization or derealization, and which may be experienced for longer than only a few minutes. Some clinical presentations of *ataque de nervios* fulfill criteria for conditions other than panic attack (e.g., other specified dissociative disorder). Also, cultural expectations may influence the classification of panic attacks as expected or unexpected, as cultural syndromes may create fear of certain situations, ranging from interpersonal arguments (associated with *ataque de nervios*), to types of exertion (associated with *khyâl* attacks), to atmospheric wind (associated with *trúng gió* attacks). Clarification of the details of cultural attributions may aid in distinguishing expected and unexpected panic attacks. For more information about cultural syndromes, see "Glossary of Cultural Concepts of Distress" in the Appendix to this manual [in DSM-5].

Gender-Related Diagnostic Issues

Panic attacks are more common in females than in males, but clinical features or symptoms of panic attacks do not differ between males and females.

Diagnostic Markers

Physiological recordings of naturally occurring panic attacks in individuals with panic disorder indicate abrupt surges of arousal, usually of heart rate, that reach a peak within minutes and subside within minutes, and for a proportion of these individuals the panic attack may be preceded by cardiorespiratory instabilities.

Functional Consequences of Panic Attacks

In the context of co-occurring mental disorders, including anxiety disorders, depressive disorders, bipolar disorder, substance use disorders, psychotic disorders, and personality disorders, panic attacks are associated with increased symptom severity, higher rates of comorbidity and suicidality, and poorer treatment response. Also, full-symptom panic attacks typically are associated with greater morbidity (e.g., greater health care utilization, more disability, poorer quality of life) than limited-symptom attacks.

Differential Diagnosis

Other paroxysmal episodes (e.g., "anger attacks").   Panic attacks should not be diagnosed if the episodes do not involve the essential feature of an abrupt surge of intense fear or intense discomfort, but rather other emotional states (e.g., anger, grief).

Anxiety disorder due to another medical condition.   Medical conditions that can cause or be misdiagnosed as panic attacks include hyperthyroidism, hyperparathyroidism, pheochromocytoma, vestibular dysfunctions, seizure disorders, and cardiopulmonary conditions (e.g., arrhythmias, supraventricular tachycardia, asthma, chronic obstructive pulmonary disease). Appropriate laboratory tests (e.g., serum calcium levels for hyperparathyroidism; Holter monitor for arrhythmias) or physical examinations (e.g., for cardiac conditions) may be helpful in determining the etiological role of another medical condition.

Substance/medication-induced anxiety disorder.   Intoxication with central nervous system stimulants (e.g., cocaine, amphetamines, caffeine) or cannabis and withdrawal from central nervous system depressants (e.g., alcohol, barbiturates) can precipitate a panic attack. A detailed history should be taken to determine if the individual had panic attacks prior to excessive substance use. Features such as onset after age 45 years or the presence of atypical symptoms during a panic attack (e.g., vertigo, loss of consciousness, loss of bladder or bowel control, slurred speech, or amnesia) suggest the possibility that a medical condition or a substance may be causing the panic attack symptoms.

Panic disorder. Repeated unexpected panic attacks are required but are not sufficient for the diagnosis of panic disorder (i.e., full diagnostic criteria for panic disorder must be met).

Comorbidity

Panic attacks are associated with increased likelihood of various comorbid mental disorders, including anxiety disorders, depressive disorders, bipolar disorders, impulse-control disorders, and substance use disorders. Panic attacks are associated with increased likelihood of later developing anxiety disorders, depressive disorders, bipolar disorders, and possibly other disorders.

Agoraphobia

Diagnostic Criteria   **300.22 (F40.00)**

A. Marked fear or anxiety about two (or more) of the following five situations:

1. Using public transportation (e.g., automobiles, buses, trains, ships, planes).
2. Being in open spaces (e.g., parking lots, marketplaces, bridges).
3. Being in enclosed places (e.g., shops, theaters, cinemas).
4. Standing in line or being in a crowd.
5. Being outside of the home alone.

B. The individual fears or avoids these situations because of thoughts that escape might be difficult or help might not be available in the event of developing panic-like symptoms or other incapacitating or embarrassing symptoms (e.g., fear of falling in the elderly; fear of incontinence).

C. The agoraphobic situations almost always provoke fear or anxiety.

D. The agoraphobic situations are actively avoided, require the presence of a companion, or are endured with intense fear or anxiety.

E. The fear or anxiety is out of proportion to the actual danger posed by the agoraphobic situations and to the sociocultural context.

F. The fear, anxiety, or avoidance is persistent, typically lasting for 6 months or more.

G. The fear, anxiety, or avoidance causes clinically significant distress or impairment in social, occupational, or other important areas of functioning.

H. If another medical condition (e.g., inflammatory bowel disease, Parkinson's disease) is present, the fear, anxiety, or avoidance is clearly excessive.

I. The fear, anxiety, or avoidance is not better explained by the symptoms of another mental disorder—for example, the symptoms are not confined to specific phobia, situational type; do not involve only social situations (as in social anxiety disorder); and are not related exclusively to obsessions (as in obsessive-compulsive disorder), perceived defects or flaws in physical appearance (as in body dysmorphic disorder), reminders of traumatic events (as in posttraumatic stress disorder), or fear of separation (as in separation anxiety disorder).

Note: Agoraphobia is diagnosed irrespective of the presence of panic disorder. If an individual's presentation meets criteria for panic disorder and agoraphobia, both diagnoses should be assigned.

Diagnostic Features

The essential feature of agoraphobia is marked, or intense, fear or anxiety triggered by the real or anticipated exposure to a wide range of situations (Criterion A). The diagnosis requires endorsement of symptoms occurring in at least two of the following five situations: 1) using public transportation, such as automobiles, buses, trains, ships, or planes; 2) being in open spaces, such as parking lots, marketplaces, or bridges; 3) being in enclosed spaces, such as shops, theaters, or cinemas; 4) standing in line or being in a crowd; or 5) being outside of the home alone. The examples for each situation are not exhaustive; other situations may be feared. When experiencing fear and anxiety cued by such situations, individuals typically experience thoughts that something terrible might happen (Criterion B). Individuals frequently believe that escape from such situations might be difficult (e.g., "can't get out of here") or that help might be unavailable (e.g., "there is nobody to help me") when panic-like symptoms or other incapacitating or embarrassing symptoms occur. "Panic-like symptoms" refer to any of the 13 symptoms included in the criteria for panic attack, such as dizziness, faintness, and fear of dying. "Other incapacitating or embarrassing symptoms" include symptoms such as vomiting and inflammatory bowel symptoms, as well as, in older adults, a fear of falling or, in children, a sense of disorientation and getting lost.

The amount of fear experienced may vary with proximity to the feared situation and may occur in anticipation of or in the actual presence of the agoraphobic situation. Also, the fear or anxiety may take the form of a full- or limited-symptom panic attack (i.e., an expected panic attack). Fear or anxiety is evoked nearly every time the individual comes into contact with the feared situation (Criterion C). Thus, an individual who becomes anxious only occasionally in an agoraphobic situation (e.g., becomes anxious when standing in line on only one out of every five occasions) would not be diagnosed with agoraphobia. The individual actively avoids the situation or, if he or she either is unable or decides not to avoid it, the situation evokes intense fear or anxiety (Criterion D). *Active avoidance* means the individual is currently behaving in ways that are intentionally designed to prevent or minimize contact with agoraphobic situations. Avoidance can be behavioral (e.g., changing daily routines, choosing a job nearby to avoid using public transportation, arranging for food delivery to avoid entering shops and supermarkets) as well as cognitive (e.g., using distraction to get through agoraphobic situations) in nature. The avoidance can become so severe that the person is completely homebound. Often, an individual is better able to confront a feared situation when accompanied by a companion, such as a partner, friend, or health professional.

The fear, anxiety, or avoidance must be out of proportion to the actual danger posed by the agoraphobic situations and to the sociocultural context (Criterion E). Differentiating clinically significant agoraphobic fears from reasonable fears (e.g., leaving the house during a bad storm) or from situations that are deemed dangerous (e.g., walking in a parking lot or using public transportation in a high-crime area) is important for a number of reasons. First, what constitutes avoidance may be difficult to judge across cultures and sociocultural contexts (e.g., it is socioculturally appropriate for orthodox Muslim women in certain parts of the world to avoid leaving the house alone, and thus such avoidance would not be considered indicative of agoraphobia). Second, older adults are likely to overattribute their fears to age-related constraints and are less likely to judge their fears as being out of proportion to the actual risk. Third, individuals with agoraphobia are likely to overestimate danger in relation to panic-like or other bodily symptoms. Agoraphobia should be diagnosed only if the fear, anxiety, or avoidance persists (Criterion F) and if it causes clinically significant distress or impairment in social, occupational, or other important areas of functioning (Criterion G). The duration of "typically lasting for 6 months or more" is meant to exclude individuals with short-lived, transient problems. However, the duration criterion should be used as a general guide, with allowance for some degree of flexibility.

Associated Features Supporting Diagnosis

In its most severe forms, agoraphobia can cause individuals to become completely homebound, unable to leave their home and dependent on others for services or assistance to provide even for basic needs. Demoralization and depressive symptoms, as well as abuse of alcohol and sedative medication as inappropriate self-medication strategies, are common.

Prevalence

Every year approximately 1.7% of adolescents and adults have a diagnosis of agoraphobia. Females are twice as likely as males to experience agoraphobia. Agoraphobia may occur in childhood, but incidence peaks in late adolescence and early adulthood. Twelve-month prevalence in individuals older than 65 years is 0.4%. Prevalence rates do not appear to vary systematically across cultural/racial groups.

Development and Course

The percentage of individuals with agoraphobia reporting panic attacks or panic disorder preceding the onset of agoraphobia ranges from 30% in community samples to more than 50% in clinic samples. The majority of individuals with panic disorder show signs of anxiety and agoraphobia before the onset of panic disorder.

In two-thirds of all cases of agoraphobia, initial onset is before age 35 years. There is a substantial incidence risk in late adolescence and early adulthood, with indications for a second high incidence risk phase after age 40 years. First onset in childhood is rare. The overall mean age at onset for agoraphobia is 17 years, although the age at onset without preceding panic attacks or panic disorder is 25–29 years.

The course of agoraphobia is typically persistent and chronic. Complete remission is rare (10%), unless the agoraphobia is treated. With more severe agoraphobia, rates of full remission decrease, whereas rates of relapse and chronicity increase. A range of other disorders, in particular other anxiety disorders, depressive disorders, substance use disorders, and personality disorders, may complicate the course of agoraphobia. The long-term course and outcome of agoraphobia are associated with substantially elevated risk of secondary major depressive disorder, persistent depressive disorder (dysthymia), and substance use disorders.

The clinical features of agoraphobia are relatively consistent across the lifespan, although the type of agoraphobic situations triggering fear, anxiety, or avoidance, as well as the type of cognitions, may vary. For example, in children, being outside of the home alone is the most frequent situation feared, whereas in older adults, being in shops, standing in line, and being in open spaces are most often feared. Also, cognitions often pertain to becoming lost (in children), to experiencing panic-like symptoms (in adults), to falling (in older adults).

The low prevalence of agoraphobia in children could reflect difficulties in symptom reporting, and thus assessments in young children may require solicitation of information from multiple sources, including parents or teachers. Adolescents, particularly males, may be less willing than adults to openly discuss agoraphobic fears and avoidance; however, agoraphobia can occur prior to adulthood and should be assessed in children and adolescents. In older adults, comorbid somatic symptom disorders, as well as motor disturbances (e.g., sense of falling or having medical complications), are frequently mentioned by individuals as the reason for their fear and avoidance. In these instances, care is to be taken in evaluating whether the fear and avoidance are out of proportion to the real danger involved.

Risk and Prognostic Factors

Temperamental.   Behavioral inhibition and neurotic disposition (i.e., negative affectivity [neuroticism] and anxiety sensitivity) are closely associated with agoraphobia but are relevant to most anxiety disorders (phobic disorders, panic disorder, generalized anxiety disorder). Anxiety sensitivity (the disposition to believe that symptoms of anxiety are harmful) is also characteristic of individuals with agoraphobia.

Environmental.   Negative events in childhood (e.g., separation, death of parent) and other stressful events, such as being attacked or mugged, are associated with the onset of agoraphobia. Furthermore, individuals with agoraphobia describe the family climate and child-rearing behavior as being characterized by reduced warmth and increased overprotection.

Genetic and physiological.   Heritability for agoraphobia is 61%. Of the various phobias, agoraphobia has the strongest and most specific association with the genetic factor that represents proneness to phobias.

Gender-Related Diagnostic Issues

Females have different patterns of comorbid disorders than males. Consistent with gender differences in the prevalence of mental disorders, males have higher rates of comorbid substance use disorders.

Functional Consequences of Agoraphobia

Agoraphobia is associated with considerable impairment and disability in terms of role functioning, work productivity, and disability days. Agoraphobia severity is a strong determinant of the degree of disability, irrespective of the presence of comorbid panic disorder, panic attacks, and other comorbid conditions. More than one-third of individuals with agoraphobia are completely homebound and unable to work.

Differential Diagnosis

When diagnostic criteria for agoraphobia and another disorder are fully met, both diagnoses should be assigned, unless the fear, anxiety, or avoidance of agoraphobia is attributable to the other disorder. Weighting of criteria and clinical judgment may be helpful in some cases.

Specific phobia, situational type.   Differentiating agoraphobia from situational specific phobia can be challenging in some cases, because these conditions share several symptom characteristics and criteria. Specific phobia, situational type, should be diagnosed versus agoraphobia if the fear, anxiety, or avoidance is limited to one of the agoraphobic situations. Requiring fears from two or more of the agoraphobic situations is a robust means for differentiating agoraphobia from specific phobias, particularly the situational subtype. Additional differentiating features include the cognitive ideation. Thus, if the situation is feared for reasons other than panic-like symptoms or other incapacitating or embarrassing symptoms (e.g., fears of being directly harmed by the situation itself, such as fear of the plane crashing for individuals who fear flying), then a diagnosis of specific phobia may be more appropriate.

Separation anxiety disorder.   Separation anxiety disorder can be best differentiated from agoraphobia by examining cognitive ideation. In separation anxiety disorder, the thoughts are about detachment from significant others and the home environment (i.e., parents or other attachment figures), whereas in agoraphobia the focus is on panic-like symptoms or other incapacitating or embarrassing symptoms in the feared situations.

Social anxiety disorder (social phobia).   Agoraphobia should be differentiated from social anxiety disorder based primarily on the situational clusters that trigger fear, anxiety, or avoidance and the cognitive ideation. In social anxiety disorder, the focus is on fear of being negatively evaluated.

Panic disorder.   When criteria for panic disorder are met, agoraphobia should not be diagnosed if the avoidance behaviors associated with the panic attacks do not extend to avoidance of two or more agoraphobic situations.

Acute stress disorder and posttraumatic stress disorder.   Acute stress disorder and PTSD can be differentiated from agoraphobia by examining whether the fear, anxiety, or avoidance is related only to situations that remind the individual of a traumatic event. If the fear, anxiety, or avoidance is restricted to trauma reminders, and if the avoidance behavior does not extend to two or more agoraphobic situations, then a diagnosis of agoraphobia is not warranted.

Major depressive disorder.   In major depressive disorder, the individual may avoid leaving home because of apathy, loss of energy, low self-esteem, and anhedonia. If the avoidance is unrelated to fears of panic-like or other incapacitating or embarrassing symptoms, then agoraphobia should not be diagnosed.

Other medical conditions.   Agoraphobia is not diagnosed if the avoidance of situations is judged to be a physiological consequence of a medical condition. This determination is based on history, laboratory findings, and a physical examination.

Other relevant medical conditions may include neurodegenerative disorders with associated motor disturbances (e.g., Parkinson's disease, multiple sclerosis), as well as cardiovascular disorders. Individuals with certain medical conditions may avoid situations because of realistic concerns about being incapacitated (e.g., fainting in an individual with transient ischemic attacks) or being embarrassed (e.g., diarrhea in an individual with Crohn's disease). The diagnosis of agoraphobia should be given only when the fear or avoidance is clearly in excess of that usually associated with these medical conditions.

Comorbidity

The majority of individuals with agoraphobia also have other mental disorders. The most frequent additional diagnoses are other anxiety disorders (e.g., specific phobias, panic disorder, social anxiety disorder), depressive disorders (major depressive disorder), PTSD, and alcohol use disorder. Whereas other anxiety disorders (e.g., separation anxiety disorder, specific phobias, panic disorder) frequently precede onset of agoraphobia, depressive disorders and substance use disorders typically occur secondary to agoraphobia.

Generalized Anxiety Disorder

Diagnostic Criteria   **300.02 (F41.1)**

A. Excessive anxiety and worry (apprehensive expectation), occurring more days than not for at least 6 months, about a number of events or activities (such as work or school performance).
B. The individual finds it difficult to control the worry.
C. The anxiety and worry are associated with three (or more) of the following six symptoms (with at least some symptoms having been present for more days than not for the past 6 months):

Note: Only one item is required in children.

1. Restlessness or feeling keyed up or on edge.
2. Being easily fatigued.
3. Difficulty concentrating or mind going blank.
4. Irritability.
5. Muscle tension.
6. Sleep disturbance (difficulty falling or staying asleep, or restless, unsatisfying sleep).

D. The anxiety, worry, or physical symptoms cause clinically significant distress or impairment in social, occupational, or other important areas of functioning.
E. The disturbance is not attributable to the physiological effects of a substance (e.g., a drug of abuse, a medication) or another medical condition (e.g., hyperthyroidism).
F. The disturbance is not better explained by another mental disorder (e.g., anxiety or worry about having panic attacks in panic disorder, negative evaluation in social anxiety disorder [social phobia], contamination or other obsessions in obsessive-compulsive disorder, separation from attachment figures in separation anxiety dis-

order, reminders of traumatic events in posttraumatic stress disorder, gaining weight in anorexia nervosa, physical complaints in somatic symptom disorder, perceived appearance flaws in body dysmorphic disorder, having a serious illness in illness anxiety disorder, or the content of delusional beliefs in schizophrenia or delusional disorder).

Diagnostic Features

The essential feature of generalized anxiety disorder is excessive anxiety and worry (apprehensive expectation) about a number of events or activities. The intensity, duration, or frequency of the anxiety and worry is out of proportion to the actual likelihood or impact of the anticipated event. The individual finds it difficult to control the worry and to keep worrisome thoughts from interfering with attention to tasks at hand. Adults with generalized anxiety disorder often worry about everyday, routine life circumstances, such as possible job responsibilities, health and finances, the health of family members, misfortune to their children, or minor matters (e.g., doing household chores or being late for appointments). Children with generalized anxiety disorder tend to worry excessively about their competence or the quality of their performance. During the course of the disorder, the focus of worry may shift from one concern to another.

Several features distinguish generalized anxiety disorder from nonpathological anxiety. First, the worries associated with generalized anxiety disorder are excessive and typically interfere significantly with psychosocial functioning, whereas the worries of everyday life are not excessive and are perceived as more manageable and may be put off when more pressing matters arise. Second, the worries associated with generalized anxiety disorder are more pervasive, pronounced, and distressing; have longer duration; and frequently occur without precipitants. The greater the range of life circumstances about which a person worries (e.g., finances, children's safety, job performance), the more likely his or her symptoms are to meet criteria for generalized anxiety disorder. Third, everyday worries are much less likely to be accompanied by physical symptoms (e.g., restlessness or feeling keyed up or on edge). Individuals with generalized anxiety disorder report subjective distress due to constant worry and related impairment in social, occupational, or other important areas of functioning.

The anxiety and worry are accompanied by at least three of the following additional symptoms: restlessness or feeling keyed up or on edge, being easily fatigued, difficulty concentrating or mind going blank, irritability, muscle tension, and disturbed sleep, although only one additional symptom is required in children.

Associated Features Supporting Diagnosis

Associated with muscle tension, there may be trembling, twitching, feeling shaky, and muscle aches or soreness. Many individuals with generalized anxiety disorder also experience somatic symptoms (e.g., sweating, nausea, diarrhea) and an exaggerated startle response. Symptoms of autonomic hyperarousal (e.g., accelerated heart rate, shortness of breath, dizziness) are less prominent in generalized anxiety disorder than in other anxiety disorders, such as panic disorder. Other conditions that may be associated with stress (e.g., irritable bowel syndrome, headaches) frequently accompany generalized anxiety disorder.

Prevalence

The 12-month prevalence of generalized anxiety disorder is 0.9% among adolescents and 2.9% among adults in the general community of the United States. The 12-month prevalence for the disorder in other countries ranges from 0.4% to 3.6%. The lifetime morbid risk is 9.0%. Females are twice as likely as males to experience generalized anxiety disorder. The prevalence of the diagnosis peaks in middle age and declines across the later years of life.

Individuals of European descent tend to experience generalized anxiety disorder more frequently than do individuals of non-European descent (i.e., Asian, African, Native American and Pacific Islander). Furthermore, individuals from developed countries are more likely than individuals from nondeveloped countries to report that they have experienced symptoms that meet criteria for generalized anxiety disorder in their lifetime.

Development and Course

Many individuals with generalized anxiety disorder report that they have felt anxious and nervous all of their lives. The median age at onset for generalized anxiety disorder is 30 years; however, age at onset is spread over a very broad range. The median age at onset is later than that for the other anxiety disorders. The symptoms of excessive worry and anxiety may occur early in life but are then manifested as an anxious temperament. Onset of the disorder rarely occurs prior to adolescence. The symptoms of generalized anxiety disorder tend to be chronic and wax and wane across the lifespan, fluctuating between syndromal and subsyndromal forms of the disorder. Rates of full remission are very low.

The clinical expression of generalized anxiety disorder is relatively consistent across the lifespan. The primary difference across age groups is in the content of the individual's worry. Children and adolescents tend to worry more about school and sporting performance, whereas older adults report greater concern about the well-being of family or their own physical heath. Thus, the content of an individual's worry tends to be age appropriate. Younger adults experience greater severity of symptoms than do older adults.

The earlier in life individuals have symptoms that meet criteria for generalized anxiety disorder, the more comorbidity they tend to have and the more impaired they are likely to be. The advent of chronic physical disease can be a potent issue for excessive worry in the elderly. In the frail elderly, worries about safety—and especially about falling—may limit activities. In those with early cognitive impairment, what appears to be excessive worry about, for example, the whereabouts of things is probably better regarded as realistic given the cognitive impairment.

In children and adolescents with generalized anxiety disorder, the anxieties and worries often concern the quality of their performance or competence at school or in sporting events, even when their performance is not being evaluated by others. There may be excessive concerns about punctuality. They may also worry about catastrophic events, such as earthquakes or nuclear war. Children with the disorder may be overly conforming, perfectionist, and unsure of themselves and tend to redo tasks because of excessive dissatisfaction with less-than-perfect performance. They are typically overzealous in seeking reassurance and approval and require excessive reassurance about their performance and other things they are worried about.

Generalized anxiety disorder may be overdiagnosed in children. When this diagnosis is being considered in children, a thorough evaluation for the presence of other childhood anxiety disorders and other mental disorders should be done to determine whether the worries may be better explained by one of these disorders. Separation anxiety disorder, social anxiety disorder (social phobia), and obsessive-compulsive disorder are often accompanied by worries that may mimic those described in generalized anxiety disorder. For example, a child with social anxiety disorder may be concerned about school performance because of fear of humiliation. Worries about illness may also be better explained by separation anxiety disorder or obsessive-compulsive disorder.

Risk and Prognostic Factors

Temperamental.   Behavioral inhibition, negative affectivity (neuroticism), and harm avoidance have been associated with generalized anxiety disorder.

Environmental.   Although childhood adversities and parental overprotection have been associated with generalized anxiety disorder, no environmental factors have been identified as specific to generalized anxiety disorder or necessary or sufficient for making the diagnosis.

Genetic and physiological.   One-third of the risk of experiencing generalized anxiety disorder is genetic, and these genetic factors overlap with the risk of neuroticism and are shared with other anxiety and mood disorders, particularly major depressive disorder.

Culture-Related Diagnostic Issues

There is considerable cultural variation in the expression of generalized anxiety disorder. For example, in some cultures, somatic symptoms predominate in the expression of the disorder, whereas in other cultures cognitive symptoms tend to predominate. This difference may be more evident on initial presentation than subsequently, as more symptoms are reported over time. There is no information as to whether the propensity for excessive worrying is related to culture, although the topic being worried about can be culture specific. It is important to consider the social and cultural context when evaluating whether worries about certain situations are excessive.

Gender-Related Diagnostic Issues

In clinical settings, generalized anxiety disorder is diagnosed somewhat more frequently in females than in males (about 55%–60% of those presenting with the disorder are female). In epidemiological studies, approximately two-thirds are female. Females and males who experience generalized anxiety disorder appear to have similar symptoms but demonstrate different patterns of comorbidity consistent with gender differences in the prevalence of disorders. In females, comorbidity is largely confined to the anxiety disorders and unipolar depression, whereas in males, comorbidity is more likely to extend to the substance use disorders as well.

Functional Consequences of Generalized Anxiety Disorder

Excessive worrying impairs the individual's capacity to do things quickly and efficiently, whether at home or at work. The worrying takes time and energy; the associated symptoms of muscle tension and feeling keyed up or on edge, tiredness, difficulty concentrating, and disturbed sleep contribute to the impairment. Importantly the excessive worrying may impair the ability of individuals with generalized anxiety disorder to encourage confidence in their children.

Generalized anxiety disorder is associated with significant disability and distress that is independent of comorbid disorders, and most non-institutionalized adults with the disorder are moderately to seriously disabled. Generalized anxiety disorder accounts for 110 million disability days per annum in the U.S. population.

Differential Diagnosis

Anxiety disorder due to another medical condition.   The diagnosis of anxiety disorder associated with another medical condition should be assigned if the individual's anxiety and worry are judged, based on history, laboratory findings, or physical examination, to be a physiological effect of another specific medical condition (e.g., pheochromocytoma, hyperthyroidism).

Substance/medication-induced anxiety disorder.   A substance/medication-induced anxiety disorder is distinguished from generalized anxiety disorder by the fact that a substance or medication (e.g., a drug of abuse, exposure to a toxin) is judged to be etiologically related to the anxiety. For example, severe anxiety that occurs only in the context of heavy coffee consumption would be diagnosed as caffeine-induced anxiety disorder.

Social anxiety disorder.   Individuals with social anxiety disorder often have anticipatory anxiety that is focused on upcoming social situations in which they must perform or be evaluated by others, whereas individuals with generalized anxiety disorder worry, whether or not they are being evaluated.

Obsessive-compulsive disorder.   Several features distinguish the excessive worry of generalized anxiety disorder from the obsessional thoughts of obsessive-compulsive disorder. In generalized anxiety disorder the focus of the worry is about forthcoming problems, and it is the excessiveness of the worry about future events that is abnormal. In obsessive-compulsive disorder, the obsessions are inappropriate ideas that take the form of intrusive and unwanted thoughts, urges, or images.

Posttraumatic stress disorder and adjustment disorders.   Anxiety is invariably present in PTSD. Generalized anxiety disorder is not diagnosed if the anxiety and worry are better explained by symptoms of PTSD. Anxiety may also be present in adjustment disorder, but this residual category should be used only when the criteria are not met for any other disorder (including generalized anxiety disorder). Moreover, in adjustment disorders, the anxiety occurs in response to an identifiable stressor within 3 months of the onset of the stressor and does not persist for more than 6 months after the termination of the stressor or its consequences.

Depressive, bipolar, and psychotic disorders.   Generalized anxiety/worry is a common associated feature of depressive, bipolar, and psychotic disorders and should not be diagnosed separately if the excessive worry has occurred only during the course of these conditions.

Comorbidity

Individuals whose presentation meets criteria for generalized anxiety disorder are likely to have met, or currently meet, criteria for other anxiety and unipolar depressive disorders. The neuroticism or emotional liability that underpins this pattern of comorbidity is associated with temperamental antecedents and genetic and environmental risk factors shared between these disorders, although independent pathways are also possible. Comorbidity with substance use, conduct, psychotic, neurodevelopmental, and neurocognitive disorders is less common.

Substance/Medication-Induced Anxiety Disorder

Diagnostic Criteria

A. Panic attacks or anxiety is predominant in the clinical picture.
B. There is evidence from the history, physical examination, or laboratory findings of both (1) and (2):
   1. The symptoms in Criterion A developed during or soon after substance intoxication or withdrawal or after exposure to a medication.
   2. The involved substance/medication is capable of producing the symptoms in Criterion A.
C. The disturbance is not better explained by an anxiety disorder that is not substance/medication-induced. Such evidence of an independent anxiety disorder could include the following:

   The symptoms precede the onset of the substance/medication use; the symptoms persist for a substantial period of time (e.g., about 1 month) after the cessation of acute withdrawal or severe intoxication; or there is other evidence suggesting the existence of an independent non-substance/medication-induced anxiety disorder (e.g., a history of recurrent non-substance/medication-related episodes).

D. The disturbance does not occur exclusively during the course of a delirium.
E. The disturbance causes clinically significant distress or impairment in social, occupational, or other important areas of functioning.

Note: This diagnosis should be made instead of a diagnosis of substance intoxication or substance withdrawal only when the symptoms in Criterion A predominate in the clinical picture and they are sufficiently severe to warrant clinical attention.

Coding note: The ICD-9-CM and ICD-10-CM codes for the [specific substance/medication]-induced anxiety disorders are indicated in the table below. Note that the ICD-10-CM code depends on whether or not there is a comorbid substance use disorder present for the same class of substance. If a mild substance use disorder is co-morbid with the substance-induced anxiety disorder, the 4th position character is "1," and the clinician should record "mild [substance] use disorder" before the substance-induced anxiety disorder (e.g., "mild cocaine use disorder with cocaine-induced anxiety disorder"). If a moderate or severe substance use disorder is comorbid with the substance-induced anxiety disorder, the 4th position character is "2," and the clinician should record "moderate [substance] use disorder" or "severe [substance] use disorder," depending on the severity of the comorbid substance use disorder. If there is no comorbid substance use disorder (e.g., after a one-time heavy use of the substance), then the 4th position character is "9," and the clinician should record only the substance-induced anxiety disorder.

		ICD-10-CM		
	ICD-9-CM	With use disorder, mild	With use disorder, moderate or severe	Without use disorder
Alcohol	291.89	F10.180	F10.280	F10.980
Caffeine	292.89	F15.180	F15.280	F15.980
Cannabis	292.89	F12.180	F12.280	F12.980
Phencyclidine	292.89	F16.180	F16.280	F16.980
Other hallucinogen	292.89	F16.180	F16.280	F16.980
Inhalant	292.89	F18.180	F18.280	F18.980
Opioid	292.89	F11.188	F11.288	F11.988
Sedative, hypnotic, or anxiolytic	292.89	F13.180	F13.280	F13.980
Amphetamine (or other stimulant)	292.89	F15.180	F15.280	F15.980
Cocaine	292.89	F14.180	F14.280	F14.980
Other (or unknown) substance	292.89	F19.180	F19.280	F19.980

Specify if (see Table 1 in the chapter "Substance-Related and Addictive Disorders" [in DSM-5] for diagnoses associated with substance class):
With onset during intoxication: This specifier applies if criteria are met for intoxication with the substance and the symptoms develop during intoxication.
With onset during withdrawal: This specifier applies if criteria are met for withdrawal from the substance and the symptoms develop during, or shortly after, withdrawal.
With onset after medication use: Symptoms may appear either at initiation of medication or after a modification or change in use.

Recording Procedures

ICD-9-CM. The name of the substance/medication-induced anxiety disorder begins with the specific substance (e.g., cocaine, salbutamol) that is presumed to be causing the anxiety symptoms. The diagnostic code is selected from the table included in the criteria set, which is based on the drug class. For substances that do not fit into any of the classes (e.g., salbutamol), the code for "other substance" should be used; and in cases in which a substance is judged to be an etiological factor but the specific class of substance is unknown, the category "unknown substance" should be used.

The name of the disorder is followed by the specification of onset (i.e., onset during intoxication, onset during withdrawal, with onset during medication use). Unlike the recording procedures for ICD-10-CM, which combine the substance-induced disorder and substance use disorder into a single code, for ICD-9-CM a separate diagnostic code is given for the substance use disorder. For example, in the case of anxiety symptoms occurring during withdrawal in a man with a severe lorazepam use disorder, the diagnosis is 292.89 lorazepam-induced anxiety disorder, with onset during withdrawal. An additional diagnosis of 304.10 severe lorazepam use disorder is also given. When more than one substance is judged to play a significant role in the development of anxiety symptoms, each should be listed separately (e.g., 292.89 methylphenidate-induced anxiety disorder, with onset during intoxication; 292.89 salbutamol-induced anxiety disorder, with onset after medication use).

ICD-10-CM.   The name of the substance/medication-induced anxiety disorder begins with the specific substance (e.g., cocaine, salbutamol) that is presumed to be causing the anxiety symptoms. The diagnostic code is selected from the table included in the criteria set, which is based on the drug class and presence or absence of a comorbid substance use disorder. For substances that do not fit into any of the classes (e.g., salbutamol), the code for "other substance" should be used; and in cases in which a substance is judged to be an etiological factor but the specific class of substance is unknown, the category "unknown substance" should be used.

When recording the name of the disorder, the comorbid substance use disorder (if any) is listed first, followed by the word "with," followed by the name of the substance-induced anxiety disorder, followed by the specification of onset (i.e., onset during intoxication, onset during withdrawal, with onset during medication use). For example, in the case of anxiety symptoms occurring during withdrawal in a man with a severe lorazepam use disorder, the diagnosis is F13.280 severe lorazepam use disorder with lorazepam-induced anxiety disorder, with onset during withdrawal. A separate diagnosis of the comorbid severe lorazepam use disorder is not given. If the substance-induced anxiety disorder occurs without a comorbid substance use disorder (e.g., after a one-time heavy use of the substance), no accompanying substance use disorder is noted (e.g., F16.980 psilocybin-induced anxiety disorder, with onset during intoxication). When more than one substance is judged to play a significant role in the development of anxiety symptoms, each should be listed separately (e.g., F15.280 severe methylphenidate use disorder with methylphenidate-induced anxiety disorder, with onset during intoxication; F19.980 salbutamol-induced anxiety disorder, with onset after medication use).

Diagnostic Features

The essential features of substance/medication-induced anxiety disorder are prominent symptoms of panic or anxiety (Criterion A) that are judged to be due to the effects of a substance (e.g., a drug of abuse, a medication, or a toxin exposure). The panic or anxiety symptoms must have developed during or soon after substance intoxication or withdrawal or after exposure to a medication, and the substances or medications must be capable of producing the symptoms (Criterion B2). Substance/medication-induced anxiety disorder due to a prescribed treatment for a mental disorder or another medical condition must have its onset while the individual is receiving the medication (or during withdrawal, if a withdrawal is associated with the medication). Once the treatment is discontinued, the panic or anxiety symptoms will usually improve or remit within days to several weeks to a month (depending on the half-life of the substance/medication and the presence of withdrawal). The diagnosis of substance/medication-induced anxiety disorder should not be given if the onset of the panic or anxiety symptoms precedes the substance/medication intoxication or withdrawal, or if the symptoms persist for a substantial period of time (i.e., usually longer than 1 month) from the time of severe intoxication or withdrawal. If the panic or anxiety symptoms persist for substantial periods of time, other causes for the symptoms should be considered.

The substance/medication-induced anxiety disorder diagnosis should be made instead of a diagnosis of substance intoxication or substance withdrawal only when the symptoms in Criterion A are predominant in the clinical picture and are sufficiently severe to warrant independent clinical attention.

Associated Features Supporting Diagnosis

Panic or anxiety can occur in association with intoxication with the following classes of substances: alcohol, caffeine, cannabis, phencyclidine, other hallucinogens, inhalants, stimulants (including cocaine), and other (or unknown) substances. Panic or anxiety can occur in association with withdrawal from the following classes of substances: alcohol; opioids; sedatives, hypnotics, and anxiolytics; stimulants (including cocaine); and other (or unknown) substances. Some medications that evoke anxiety symptoms include anesthetics and analgesics, sympathomimetics or other bronchodilators, anticholinergics, insulin, thyroid preparations, oral contraceptives, antihistamines, antiparkinsonian medications, corticosteroids, antihypertensive and cardiovascular medications, anticonvulsants, lithium carbonate, antipsychotic medications, and antidepressant medications. Heavy metals and toxins (e.g., organophosphate insecticide, nerve gases, carbon monoxide, carbon dioxide, volatile substances such as gasoline and paint) may also cause panic or anxiety symptoms.

Prevalence

The prevalence of substance/medication-induced anxiety disorder is not clear. General population data suggest that it may be rare, with a 12-month prevalence of approximately 0.002%. However, in clinical populations, the prevalence is likely to be higher.

Diagnostic Markers

Laboratory assessments (e.g., urine toxicology) may be useful to measure substance intoxication as part of an assessment for substance/medication-induced anxiety disorder.

Differential Diagnosis

Substance intoxication and substance withdrawal. Anxiety symptoms commonly occur in substance intoxication and substance withdrawal. The diagnosis of the substance-specific intoxication or substance-specific withdrawal will usually suffice to categorize the symptom presentation. A diagnosis of substance/medication-induced anxiety disorder should be made in addition to substance intoxication or substance withdrawal when the panic or anxiety symptoms are predominant in the clinical picture and are sufficiently severe to warrant independent clinical attention. For example, panic or anxiety symptoms are characteristic of alcohol withdrawal.

Anxiety disorder (i.e., not induced by a substance/medication). Substance/medication-induced anxiety disorder is judged to be etiologically related to the substance/medication. Substance/medication-induced anxiety disorder is distinguished from a primary anxiety disorder based on the onset, course, and other factors with respect to substances/medications. For drugs of abuse, there must be evidence from the history, physical examination, or laboratory findings for use, intoxication, or withdrawal. Substance/medication-induced anxiety disorders arise only in association with intoxication or withdrawal states, whereas primary anxiety disorders may precede the onset of substance/medication use. The presence of features that are atypical of a primary anxiety disorder, such as atypical age at onset (e.g., onset of panic disorder after age 45 years) or symptoms (e.g., atypical panic attack symptoms such as true vertigo, loss of balance, loss of consciousness, loss of bladder control, headaches, slurred speech) may suggest a substance/medication-induced etiology. A primary anxiety disorder diagnosis is warranted if the panic or anxiety symptoms persist for a substantial period of time (about 1 month or longer) after the end of the substance intoxication or acute withdrawal or there is a history of an anxiety disorder.

Delirium. If panic or anxiety symptoms occur exclusively during the course of delirium, they are considered to be an associated feature of the delirium and are not diagnosed separately.

Anxiety disorder due to another medical condition. If the panic or anxiety symptoms are attributed to the physiological consequences of another medical condition (i.e., rather than to the medication taken for the medical condition), anxiety disorder due to another medical condition should be diagnosed. The history often provides the basis for such a judgment. At times, a change in the treatment for the other medical condition (e.g., medication substitution or discontinuation) may be needed to determine whether the medication is the causative agent (in which case the symptoms may be better explained by substance/medication-induced anxiety disorder). If the disturbance is attributable to both another medical condition and substance use, both diagnoses (i.e., anxiety disorder due to another medical condition and substance/medication-induced anxiety disorder) may be given. When there is insufficient evidence to determine whether the panic or anxiety symptoms are attributable to a substance/medication or to another medical condition or are primary (i.e., not attributable to either a substance or another medical condition), a diagnosis of other specified or unspecified anxiety disorder would be indicated.

Anxiety Disorder Due to Another Medical Condition

Diagnostic Criteria	293.84 (F06.4)

A. Panic attacks or anxiety is predominant in the clinical picture.

B. There is evidence from the history, physical examination, or laboratory findings that the disturbance is the direct pathophysiological consequence of another medical condition.

C. The disturbance is not better explained by another mental disorder.

D. The disturbance does not occur exclusively during the course of a delirium.

E. The disturbance causes clinically significant distress or impairment in social, occupational, or other important areas of functioning.

Coding note: Include the name of the other medical condition within the name of the mental disorder (e.g., 293.84 [F06.4] anxiety disorder due to pheochromocytoma). The other medical condition should be coded and listed separately immediately before the anxiety disorder due to the medical condition (e.g., 227.0 [D35.00] pheochromocytoma; 293.84 [F06.4] anxiety disorder due to pheochromocytoma.

Diagnostic Features

The essential feature of anxiety disorder due to another medical condition is clinically significant anxiety that is judged to be best explained as a physiological effect of another medical condition. Symptoms can include prominent anxiety symptoms or panic attacks (Criterion A). The judgment that the symptoms are best explained by the associated physical condition must be based on evidence from the history, physical examination, or laboratory findings (Criterion B). Additionally, it must be judged that the symptoms are not better accounted for by another mental disorder, in particular, adjustment disorder, with anxiety, in which the stressor is the medical condition (Criterion C). In this case, an individual with adjustment disorder is especially distressed about the meaning or the consequences of the associated medical condition. By contrast, there is often a prominent physical component to the anxiety (e.g., shortness of breath) when the anxiety is due to another medical condition. The diagnosis is not made if the anxiety symptoms occur only during the course of a delirium (Criterion D). The anxiety symptoms must cause clinically significant distress or impairment in social, occupational, or other important areas of functioning (Criterion E).

In determining whether the anxiety symptoms are attributable to another medical condition, the clinician must first establish the presence of the medical condition. Furthermore, it must be established that anxiety symptoms can be etiologically related to the medical condition through a physiological mechanism before making a judgment that this is the best explanation for the symptoms in a specific individual. A careful and comprehensive assessment of multiple factors is necessary to make this judgment. Several aspects of the clinical presentation should be considered: 1) the presence of a clear temporal association between the onset, exacerbation, or remission of the medical condition and the anxiety symptoms; 2) the presence of features that are atypical of a primary anxiety disorder (e.g., atypical age at onset or course); and 3) evidence in the literature that a known physiological mechanism (e.g., hyperthyroidism) causes anxiety. In addition, the disturbance must not be better explained by a primary anxiety disorder, a substance/medication-induced anxiety disorder, or another primary mental disorder (e.g., adjustment disorder).

Associated Features Supporting Diagnosis

A number of medical conditions are known to include anxiety as a symptomatic manifestation. Examples include endocrine disease (e.g., hyperthyroidism, pheochromocytoma, hypoglycemia, hyperadrenocortisolism), cardiovascular disorders (e.g., congestive heart failure, pulmonary embolism, arrhythmia such as atrial fibrillation), respiratory illness (e.g., chronic obstructive pulmonary disease, asthma, pneumonia), metabolic disturbances (e.g., vitamin B_{12} deficiency, porphyria), and neurological illness (e.g., neoplasms, vestibular dysfunction, encephalitis, seizure disorders). Anxiety due to another medical condition is diagnosed when the medical condition is known to induce anxiety and when the medical condition preceded the onset of the anxiety.

Prevalence

The prevalence of anxiety disorder due to another medical condition is unclear. There appears to be an elevated prevalence of anxiety disorders among individuals with a variety of medical conditions, including asthma, hypertension, ulcers, and arthritis. However, this increased prevalence may be due to reasons other than the anxiety disorder directly causing the medical condition.

Development and Course

The development and course of anxiety disorder due to another medical condition generally follows the course of the underlying illness. This diagnosis is not meant to include primary anxiety disorders that arise in the context of chronic medical illness. This is important to consider with older adults, who may experience chronic medical illness and then develop independent anxiety disorders secondary to the chronic medical illness.

Diagnostic Markers

Laboratory assessments and/or medical examinations are necessary to confirm the diagnosis of the associated medical condition.

Differential Diagnosis

Delirium. A separate diagnosis of anxiety disorder due to another medical condition is not given if the anxiety disturbance occurs exclusively during the course of a delirium. However, a diagnosis of anxiety disorder due to another medical condition may be given in addition to a diagnosis of major neurocognitive disorder (dementia) if the etiology of anxiety is judged to be a physiological consequence of the pathological process causing the neurocognitive disorder and if anxiety is a prominent part of the clinical presentation.

Mixed presentation of symptoms (e.g., mood and anxiety).   If the presentation includes a mix of different types of symptoms, the specific mental disorder due to another medical condition depends on which symptoms predominate in the clinical picture.

Substance/medication-induced anxiety disorder.   If there is evidence of recent or prolonged substance use (including medications with psychoactive effects), withdrawal from a substance, or exposure to a toxin, a substance/medication-induced anxiety disorder should be considered. Certain medications are known to increase anxiety (e.g., corticosteroids, estrogens, metoclopramide), and when this is the case, the medication may be the most likely etiology, although it may be difficult to distinguish whether the anxiety is attributable to the medications or to the medical illness itself. When a diagnosis of substance-induced anxiety is being made in relation to recreational or nonprescribed drugs, it may be useful to obtain a urine or blood drug screen or other appropriate laboratory evaluation. Symptoms that occur during or shortly after (i.e., within 4 weeks of) substance intoxication or withdrawal or after medication use may be especially indicative of a substance/medication-induced anxiety disorder, depending on the type, duration, or amount of the substance used. If the disturbance is associated with both another medical condition and substance use, both diagnoses (i.e., anxiety disorder due to another medical condition and substance/medication-induced anxiety disorder) can be given. Features such as onset after age 45 years or the presence of atypical symptoms during a panic attack (e.g., vertigo, loss of consciousness, loss of bladder or bowel control, slurred speech, amnesia) suggest the possibility that another medical condition or a substance may be causing the panic attack symptoms.

Anxiety disorder (not due to a known medical condition).   Anxiety disorder due to another medical condition should be distinguished from other anxiety disorders (especially panic disorder and generalized anxiety disorder). In other anxiety disorders, no specific and direct causative physiological mechanisms associated with another medical condition can be demonstrated. Late age at onset, atypical symptoms, and the absence of a personal or family history of anxiety disorders suggest the need for a thorough assessment to rule out the diagnosis of anxiety disorder due to another medical condition. Anxiety disorders can exacerbate or pose increased risk for medical conditions such as cardiovascular events and myocardial infarction and should not be diagnosed as anxiety disorder due to another medical condition in these cases.

Illness anxiety disorder.   Anxiety disorder due to another medical condition should be distinguished from illness anxiety disorder. Illness anxiety disorder is characterized by worry about illness, concern about pain, and bodily preoccupations. In the case of illness anxiety disorder, individuals may or may not have diagnosed medical conditions. Although an individual with illness anxiety disorder and a diagnosed medical condition is likely to experience anxiety about the medical condition, the medical condition is not physiologically related to the anxiety symptoms.

Adjustment disorders.   Anxiety disorder due to another medical condition should be distinguished from adjustment disorders, with anxiety, or with anxiety and depressed mood. Adjustment disorder is warranted when individuals experience a maladaptive response to the stress of having another medical condition. The reaction to stress usually concerns the meaning or consequences of the stress, as compared with the experience of anxiety or mood symptoms that occur as a physiological consequence of the other medical condition. In adjustment disorder, the anxiety symptoms are typically related to coping with the stress of having a general medical condition, whereas in anxiety disorder due to another medical condition, individuals are more likely to have prominent physical symptoms and to be focused on issues other than the stress of the illness itself.

Associated feature of another mental disorder.   Anxiety symptoms may be an associated feature of another mental disorder (e.g., schizophrenia, anorexia nervosa).

Other specified or unspecified anxiety disorder.   This diagnosis is given if it cannot be determined whether the anxiety symptoms are primary, substance-induced, or associated with another medical condition.

Other Specified Anxiety Disorder

300.09 (F41.8)

This category applies to presentations in which symptoms characteristic of an anxiety disorder that cause clinically significant distress or impairment in social, occupational, or other important areas of functioning predominate but do not meet the full criteria for any of the disorders in the anxiety disorders diagnostic class. The other specified anxiety disorder category is used in situations in which the clinician chooses to communicate the specific reason that the presentation does not meet the criteria for any specific anxiety disorder. This is done by recording "other specified anxiety disorder" followed by the specific reason (e.g., "generalized anxiety not occurring more days than not").

Examples of presentations that can be specified using the "other specified" designation include the following:

1. **Limited-symptom attacks.**
2. **Generalized anxiety not occurring more days than not.**
3. ***Khyâl cap*** **(wind attacks):** See "Glossary of Cultural Concepts of Distress" in the Appendix [in DSM-5].
4. ***Ataque de nervios*** **(attack of nerves):** See "Glossary of Cultural Concepts of Distress" in the Appendix [in DSM-5].

Unspecified Anxiety Disorder

300.00 (F41.9)

This category applies to presentations in which symptoms characteristic of an anxiety disorder that cause clinically significant distress or impairment in social, occupational, or other important areas of functioning predominate but do not meet the full criteria for any of the disorders in the anxiety disorders diagnostic class. The unspecified anxiety disorder category is used in situations in which the clinician chooses *not* to specify the reason that the criteria are not met for a specific anxiety disorder, and includes presentations in which there is insufficient information to make a more specific diagnosis (e.g., in emergency room settings).

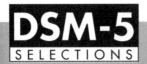

Anxiety Disorders

DSM-5® Guidebook

309.21 (F93.0)	Separation Anxiety Disorder
313.23 (F94.0)	Selective Mutism
300.29 (F40.2__)	Specific Phobia
300.23 (F40.10)	Social Anxiety Disorder (Social Phobia)
300.01 (F41.0)	Panic Disorder
	Panic Attack Specifier
300.22 (F40.00)	Agoraphobia
300.02 (F41.1)	Generalized Anxiety Disorder
	Substance/Medication-Induced Anxiety Disorder
293.84 (F06.4)	Anxiety Disorder Due to Another Medical Condition
300.09 (F41.8)	Other Specified Anxiety Disorder
300.00 (F41.9)	Unspecified Anxiety Disorder

Anxiety disorders are among the most prevalent psychiatric conditions worldwide. Research consistently shows them to be associated with increased psychiatric and physical morbidity, use of health care services, and psychosocial impairment. Necessity dictates that clinicians recognize and treat anxiety disorders without delay. Table 1 lists the DSM-5 anxiety disorders.

TABLE 1. Anxiety disorders

Separation anxiety disorder

Selective mutism

Specific phobia

Social anxiety disorder (social phobia)

Panic disorder

Agoraphobia

Generalized anxiety disorder

Substance/medication-induced anxiety disorder

Anxiety disorder due to another medical condition

Other specified anxiety disorder

Unspecified anxiety disorder

The word *anxiety* has been used to describe diverse phenomena, but in the clinical literature the term refers to the presence of fear or apprehension that is out of proportion to the situation. Anxiety was considered to play an important role in several conditions identified in the nineteenth century (Goodwin and Guze 1989). In the late nineteenth century, Da Costa wrote about an "irritable heart syndrome," characterized by chest pain, palpitations, and dizziness, a disorder thought to be due to a functional cardiac disturbance. He described the syndrome as occurring in a Civil War veteran, and later the syndrome was variously referred to as "soldier's heart," the "effort syndrome," or "neurocirculatory asthenia." At about the same time, Beard described *neurasthenia,* thought to be a disorder of nervous exhaustion. Freud later separated neurasthenia from cases affected mainly with anxiety symptoms under the name *anxiety neurosis.* He described its clinical characteristics as including general irritability, anxious expectation, pangs of conscience, anxiety attacks, and phobias.

In DSM-I, the category psychoneurotic disorders constituted a distinct class in which anxiety was the chief characteristic. According to DSM-I, the anxiety "may be directly felt and expressed or…may be unconsciously and automatically controlled by the utilization of various psychological defense mechanisms" (p. 31). Several "reactions" were enumerated, including "anxiety reaction" and "phobic reaction"—disorders that continue to be recognized as anxiety disorders—and others that now fall into separate categories (i.e., dissociative reaction, obsessive compulsive reaction). In DSM-II, the category was renamed "neuroses" and the term *reaction* was eliminated, but the category was otherwise mostly unchanged.

DSM-III's all-encompassing changes led to a regrouping of some disorders and the creation of new disorders in which anxiety was either experienced as the predominant disturbance or experienced by the person as he or she attempted to master its symptoms (e.g., confronting a dreaded object or situation). The new diagnostic class, anxiety disorders, included panic disorder, agoraphobia, social phobia, simple phobia, generalized anxiety disorder, obsessive-compulsive disorder, and post-traumatic stress disorder (which was hyphenated until DSM-IV). Acute stress disorder was later added in DSM-IV. DSM-III-R, DSM-IV, and DSM-IV-TR otherwise remained true to DSM-III, except for minor changes in the criteria sets and some name changes (e.g., from simple phobia to specific phobia).

In DSM-5, the anxiety disorders chapter has remained largely faithful to its immediate predecessor, with several major exceptions. Obsessive-compulsive disorder now has its own chapter (see Chapter 7, "Obsessive-Compulsive and Related Disorders"). Posttraumatic stress disorder and acute stress disorder have been moved to "Trauma- and Stressor-Related Disorders" (see Chapter 8). These changes were made in response to scientific data showing that these disorders stand apart from the other anxiety disorders. The sequential order of the chapters in DSM-5 (i.e., the metastructure), however, reflects the close relationship among the disorders. Last, separation anxiety disorder and selective mutism are new to the chapter, having been formerly included in the DSM-IV chapter "Disorders Usually First Diagnosed in Infancy, Childhood, or Adolescence."

Other changes include the wording of criteria sets, which have been modified to 1) reflect the dysfunction underlying these disorders as intense, frequent, and chronic fear and anxiety; 2) separate the main constructs (e.g., situational triggers, cognitive ideation, intensity, frequency, duration); and 3) enhance consistency across the disorders. For specific phobia and social anxiety disorder, changes include deletion of the requirement that adults recognize that their anxiety is excessive or unreasonable. In addition, the minimum 6-month duration, which had been limited to individuals under age 18 years in DSM-IV, has been extended to all ages. The essential features of panic attacks remain unchanged, but the terminology for describing different types has been replaced with the terms *expected* or *unexpected*. Panic disorder and agoraphobia have been unlinked, and the criteria for agoraphobia have been extended to be consistent with criteria sets for the other disorders. With social anxiety disorder, the "generalized" specifier had been deleted and replaced with a "performance only" specifier.

Separation Anxiety Disorder

Separation anxiety disorder is a condition in which a person has excessive anxiety regarding separation from places or people to whom he or she has a strong emotional attachment. Included with the childhood disorders in DSM-III through DSM-IV-TR, separation anxiety disorder has now been moved because of research that links it to the anxiety disorders and the growing recognition that it occurs in adults. In fact, the lifetime estimate of separation anxiety disorder in childhood is 4.1%, whereas the rate among adults is 6.6%. Although about one-third of adults with separation anxiety disorder had it in childhood, the majority of adults had a first onset in adulthood. In children, the strong emotional attachment is likely to a parent; with adults, the attachment might be to a spouse or a friend.

Separation anxiety disorder should not be confused with separation anxiety that occurs as a normal stage of development for healthy, secure babies. Separation anxiety typically starts at around 8 months of age and increases until 13–15 months, when it begins to decline.

Diagnostic Criteria for Separation Anxiety Disorder　　**309.21 (F93.0)**

A. Developmentally inappropriate and excessive fear or anxiety concerning separation from those to whom the individual is attached, as evidenced by at least three of the following:

1. Recurrent excessive distress when anticipating or experiencing separation from home or from major attachment figures.
2. Persistent and excessive worry about losing major attachment figures or about possible harm to them, such as illness, injury, disasters, or death.
3. Persistent and excessive worry about experiencing an untoward event (e.g., getting lost, being kidnapped, having an accident, becoming ill) that causes separation from a major attachment figure.
4. Persistent reluctance or refusal to go out, away from home, to school, to work, or elsewhere because of fear of separation.
5. Persistent and excessive fear of or reluctance about being alone or without major attachment figures at home or in other settings.

6. Persistent reluctance or refusal to sleep away from home or to go to sleep without being near a major attachment figure.
7. Repeated nightmares involving the theme of separation.
8. Repeated complaints of physical symptoms (e.g., headaches, stomachaches, nausea, vomiting) when separation from major attachment figures occurs or is anticipated.

B. The fear, anxiety, or avoidance is persistent, lasting at least 4 weeks in children and adolescents and typically 6 months or more in adults.
C. The disturbance causes clinically significant distress or impairment in social, academic, occupational, or other important areas of functioning.
D. The disturbance is not better explained by another mental disorder, such as refusing to leave home because of excessive resistance to change in autism spectrum disorder; delusions or hallucinations concerning separation in psychotic disorders; refusal to go outside without a trusted companion in agoraphobia; worries about ill health or other harm befalling significant others in generalized anxiety disorder; or concerns about having an illness in illness anxiety disorder.

Criterion A

Although some separation anxiety is normal at various developmental phases, when the fear or anxiety is excessive and functionally impairing, this diagnosis may be appropriate. To increase the relevance to adults with separation anxiety disorder, terms have been added (e.g., addition of "work" in Criterion A4) or deleted (e.g., removal of "adults" in DSM-IV's Criterion A5 because attachment figures are not always adults; for adults, attachment figures can be partners, children, and so forth).

Criterion B

The duration is specified as typically lasting at least 6 months in adults (instead of the 4-week requirement in DSM-IV that has been retained in DSM-5 for children and adolescents) to minimize overdiagnosis of transient fears. A caveat permits shorter durations in cases of acute onset or exacerbation of severe symptoms.

Criteria C and D

Separation anxiety disorder is associated with significant impairment. People with the disorder may refuse to attend school or work, complain of somatic problems, and become socially isolated. Untreated, the disorder is associated with low educational attainment, unemployment, and either remaining unmarried or experiencing marital disruption. Because separation anxiety may occur in association with other mental disorders, the clinician needs to determine whether the person's symptoms meet full criteria for an independent diagnosis of separation anxiety disorder.

Selective Mutism

Selective mutism is characterized by the consistent failure to speak in specific social situations where speaking is expected despite being able to speak in other situations (e.g., at home). Originally named "elective mutism" in DSM-III, and renamed "selective mutism" for DSM-IV, the disorder was included with DSM-IV's "Disorders Usually First Diagnosed in Infancy, Childhood, or Adolescence." Selective mutism has been moved because of research that connects it with the anxiety disorders, and growing recognition that it continues into adulthood (or in rare cases begins in adulthood). Selective mutism is rare and most likely to manifest in young children.

Diagnostic Criteria for Selective Mutism   **313.23 (F94.0)**

A. Consistent failure to speak in specific social situations in which there is an expectation for speaking (e.g., at school) despite speaking in other situations.
B. The disturbance interferes with educational or occupational achievement or with social communication.
C. The duration of the disturbance is at least 1 month (not limited to the first month of school).
D. The failure to speak is not attributable to a lack of knowledge of, or comfort with, the spoken language required in the social situation.
E. The disturbance is not better explained by a communication disorder (e.g., childhood-onset fluency disorder) and does not occur exclusively during the course of autism spectrum disorder, schizophrenia, or another psychotic disorder.

Criterion A

When encountering individuals in specific social interactions, children and adults with selective mutism do not initiate speech or reciprocally respond when spoken to by others. These same individuals when seen at home, however, can interact normally. The diagnosis requires a *consistent* failure to speak in social situations.

Criterion B

Selective mutism is associated with significant impairment. Children with selective mutism often refuse to speak at school, leading to academic or educational impairment. As these children mature, they may face increasing social isolation, and in school settings, they suffer academic impairment because often they do not communicate appropriately with teachers regarding academic or personal needs.

Criterion C

Selective silence lasting less than a month (e.g., a child's being upset and refusing to talk for a few days) would not meet criteria for the diagnosis.

Criterion D

Children in families who have immigrated to a country where a different language is spoken may refuse to speak the new language because of lack of knowledge of the language. If comprehension of the new language is adequate but refusal to speak persists, a diagnosis of selective mutism would be warranted.

Criterion E

Although children with selective mutism generally have normal language skills, there may occasionally be an associated communication disorder. Selective mutism should be distinguished from speech disturbances that are better explained by a communication disorder, such as language disorder, speech sound disorder (previously phonological disorder), childhood-onset fluency disorder (stuttering), or pragmatic (social) communication disorder. Unlike selective mutism, the speech disturbance in these conditions is not restricted to a specific social situation. Individuals with autism spectrum disorder, schizophrenia or other psychotic disorders, or severe intellectual disability may have problems with social communication and be unable to speak appropriately in social situations. In contrast, selective mutism should be diagnosed only when a child has an established capacity to speak in some social situations (typically at home).

Specific Phobia

The term *phobia* refers to an excessive fear of a specific object, circumstance, or situation. Phobias are classified on the basis of the feared object or situation. Both specific phobia and social anxiety disorder (social phobia) require the development of intense anxiety, upon exposure to the feared object or situation. Both diagnoses also require that the fear or anxiety either interferes with functioning or causes marked distress.

Specific phobia includes the following specifiers: animal, natural environment, blood-injection-injury, situational, and other (for phobias that do not clearly fall into the previous four categories). The key feature for each stimulus type is that the fear or anxiety is limited to a specific object, both temporally and with respect to other objects. An individual with specific phobia becomes immediately frightened or anxious when presented with a feared object. This fear may relate to concern about harm from a feared object, concern about embarrassment, or fear of consequences related to exposure to the feared object. For example, individuals with blood-injection-injury phobia may be afraid of fainting on exposure to blood, and individuals with fear of heights may be afraid of becoming dizzy.

Specific phobia may involve fear of more than one object, particularly within a specific subcategory of phobia. For example, an individual with a phobia of insects may also have a phobia of mice, both phobias being classified as animal-type phobias. Quantifying the impairment associated with a specific phobia is sometimes difficult, because a comorbid disorder typically tends to cause more impairment than a specific phobia. Impairment associated with specific phobia typically restricts the social or professional activities of the individual.

Phobias have been recognized as incapacitating for more than 100 years. The prominent place of phobias in the history of modern mental health is indicated by the major role that case histories of patients with phobias played in the development of both psychoanalytic and cognitive therapies. The phobia category has undergone progressive refinement over the years. In DSM-III, phobias were regarded as a group of related but distinct conditions. Between DSM-III and DSM-IV, specific phobia was modified to include subcategories, based on research noting distinct physiology and demographics of the stimulus types.

Specific phobias are usually quite easily distinguished from other conditions because of the focused nature of the anxiety, both over time and with respect to objects or situations. The most difficult diagnostic issues involve differentiating specific phobia from other anxiety disorders.

Specific phobia exhibits a bimodal age at onset, with a childhood peak for animal phobia, natural environment phobia, and blood-injection-injury phobia and an early adulthood peak for other phobias, such as situational phobia. Because individuals with isolated specific phobias rarely present for treatment, research on the course of the disorder in the clinic is limited. Data suggest that most specific phobias that begin in childhood and persist into adulthood will continue to persist over many years. The severity of the condition when it persists into adulthood is thought to remain relatively constant, without the waxing and waning course of the disorder during childhood and adolescence or seen with other anxiety disorders.

Diagnostic Criteria for Specific Phobia

A. Marked fear or anxiety about a specific object or situation (e.g., flying, heights, animals, receiving an injection, seeing blood).

   Note: In children, the fear or anxiety may be expressed by crying, tantrums, freezing, or clinging.

B. The phobic object or situation almost always provokes immediate fear or anxiety.

C. The phobic object or situation is actively avoided or endured with intense fear or anxiety.

D. The fear or anxiety is out of proportion to the actual danger posed by the specific object or situation and to the sociocultural context.

E. The fear, anxiety, or avoidance is persistent, typically lasting for 6 months or more.

F. The fear, anxiety, or avoidance causes clinically significant distress or impairment in social, occupational, or other important areas of functioning.

G. The disturbance is not better explained by the symptoms of another mental disorder, including fear, anxiety, and avoidance of situations associated with panic-like symptoms or other incapacitating symptoms (as in agoraphobia); objects or situations related to obsessions (as in obsessive-compulsive disorder); reminders of traumatic events (as in posttraumatic stress disorder); separation from home or attachment figures (as in separation anxiety disorder); or social situations (as in social anxiety disorder).

Specify if:
   Code based on the phobic stimulus:
   300.29 (F40.218) Animal (e.g., spiders, insects, dogs).
   300.29 (F40.228) Natural environment (e.g., heights, storms, water).
   300.29 (F40.23x) Blood-injection-injury (e.g., needles, invasive medical procedures).

   > **Coding note:** Select specific ICD-10-CM code as follows: **F40.230** fear of blood; **F40.231** fear of injections and transfusions; **F40.232** fear of other medical care; or **F40.233** fear of injury.

300.29 (F40.248) Situational (e.g., airplanes, elevators, enclosed places).
300.29 (F40.298) Other (e.g., situations that may lead to choking or vomiting; in children, e.g., loud sounds or costumed characters).

Coding note: When more than one phobic stimulus is present, code all ICD-10-CM codes that apply (e.g., for fear of snakes and flying, F40.218 specific phobia, animal, and F40.248 specific phobia, situational).

Criteria A and B

There is marked fear or anxiety that is triggered by exposure to a specific stimulus. The term *marked* has been operationalized as "intense." The phrase "fear or anxiety" is used consistently across anxiety disorders. The phobic object or situation almost always provokes immediate fear or anxiety.

Criterion C

There are generally two responses to the fear or anxiety elicited by the stimulus. A person may avoid situations in which he or she is exposed to the stimulus, or the person may expose himself or herself to the phobic object or situation and endure the fear or anxiety. DSM-5 has added the descriptor "actively avoided" to minimize overdiagnosis of mild fears.

Criterion D

The fear or anxiety is out of proportion, or more intense than is deemed necessary, given the actual danger that the object or situation poses—that is, the fear or anxiety is greater than is deemed appropriate to the actual danger in the situation. Although people with specific phobia often recognize their reactions as disproportionate to the situation, they tend to overestimate the danger in their feared situations, and thus the judgment of being out of proportion should not be made solely on the basis of self-report. In DSM-IV, Criterion C required that the individual be aware that the fear or anxiety was excessive, but stated that this requirement might not be present in children. Self-recognition has been removed because many adults deny that their fears are out of proportion or excessive, and the notation that in children the feature many be absent has been deleted. This criterion requires that the sociocultural context be taken into account.

Criterion E

With the duration criterion "typically lasting for 6 months or more" (with text clarification that the cutoff should not be applied too rigidly), the overdiagnosis of transient fears and phobias should be minimized. DSM-IV included a duration criterion (6 months or more) for children under age 18, but this is now extended to all age groups given the evidence that transient fears and phobias occur in adulthood.

Criterion F

The fear, anxiety, or avoidance needs to result in clinically significant distress or functional impairment. For example, a person who avoids the ferris wheel at a state fair because of fear of heights may still have a lovely day at the fair and pay little heed to how this fear affects the experience. Some people cope with their phobias by manipulating their environments (e.g., avoidance of zoos by a person who fears snakes). In these cases, the impairment would be minimal or nonexistent and the person's presentation would not qualify for the diagnosis. If the manipulation of the environment affects the person's work, for example, then it may cause significant interference.

Criterion G

Many disorders are characterized by avoidance (e.g., obsessive-compulsive disorder, agoraphobia). Specific phobia should be diagnosed only when avoidance is related to an object or situation and is not accounted for by another disorder.

Specifiers

The specifiers reflect the general categories of phobic stimulus. DSM-5 has removed reference to fears of contracting an illness in the "other" category because of the relatedness of such fears to obsessive-compulsive disorder and to hypochondriasis (which has been replaced, in DSM-5, by somatic symptom disorder and, in a minority of cases, illness anxiety disorder).

Social Anxiety Disorder (Social Phobia)

Social anxiety disorder involves fear of or anxiety about social situations, including situations that involve scrutiny or contact with strangers. Individuals with this disorder typically fear embarrassing themselves in social situations, such as while speaking in public or meeting new people. This disorder can involve specific fears or anxiety about performing certain activities, such as writing, eating, or speaking in front of others. It can also involve a vague, nonspecific fear of embarrassing oneself or feeling foolish. The clinician should recognize that many individuals exhibit at least some social anxiety or self-consciousness. Community studies suggest that roughly one-third of all people consider themselves to be more anxious than other people in social situations. Such anxiety becomes a disorder only when the anxiety either prevents the person from participating in desired activities or causes marked distress in such activities.

Diagnostic Criteria for Social Anxiety Disorder
(Social Phobia)   **300.23** (F40.10)

A. Marked fear or anxiety about one or more social situations in which the individual is exposed to possible scrutiny by others. Examples include social interactions (e.g., having a conversation, meeting unfamiliar people), being observed (e.g., eating or drinking), and performing in front of others (e.g., giving a speech).

   Note: In children, the anxiety must occur in peer settings and not just during interactions with adults.

B. The individual fears that he or she will act in a way or show anxiety symptoms that will be negatively evaluated (i.e., will be humiliating or embarrassing; will lead to rejection or offend others).

C. The social situations almost always provoke fear or anxiety.

   Note: In children, the fear or anxiety may be expressed by crying, tantrums, freezing, clinging, shrinking, or failing to speak in social situations.

D. The social situations are avoided or endured with intense fear or anxiety.

E. The fear or anxiety is out of proportion to the actual threat posed by the social situation and to the sociocultural context.

F. The fear, anxiety, or avoidance is persistent, typically lasting for 6 months or more.

G. The fear, anxiety, or avoidance causes clinically significant distress or impairment in social, occupational, or other important areas of functioning.

H. The fear, anxiety, or avoidance is not attributable to the physiological effects of a substance (e.g., a drug of abuse, a medication) or another medical condition.

I. The fear, anxiety, or avoidance is not better explained by the symptoms of another mental disorder, such as panic disorder, body dysmorphic disorder, or autism spectrum disorder.

J. If another medical condition (e.g., Parkinson's disease, obesity, disfigurement from burns or injury) is present, the fear, anxiety, or avoidance is clearly unrelated or is excessive.

Specify if:

   Performance only: If the fear is restricted to speaking or performing in public.

Criteria A and B

These items cover the three contexts in which social anxiety disorder most commonly occurs: social interactions, being observed by others, and performing in front of others.

In Criterion B, *humiliation* and *embarrassment* have been brought under the broader phrase "negatively evaluated," which is the core fear in social anxiety disorder. The phrase "offend others" has been added to increase cultural sensitivity; in some cultures the underlying fear is the concern that one will make others uncomfortable.

Criterion C

This criterion highlights that social anxiety is a conditioned, stimulus response. In addition, the criterion clarifies that in children, fear and anxiety may present in a range of ways (e.g., tantrums).

Criterion D

Although some individuals with social anxiety disorder avoid the contexts that elicit their anxiety, others endure the anxiety-provoking environments even when the anxiety or fear is intense.

Criterion E

People with social anxiety disorder often have difficulty recognizing that their fear is excessive. Therefore, the clinician may be in a better position to judge this. Use of the phrase "out of proportion to the actual threat posed" is intended to operationalize what was meant by "excessive or unreasonable" in DSM-IV. Criterion C in DSM-IV included a note that self-recognition may be absent in children; this note has been deleted. Finally, the DSM-5 item reminds the clinician to take into account the "sociocultural context."

Criterion F

The DSM-IV requirement that the duration be 6 months or more in children under age 18 years has now been extended to all age groups, given the data that transient social anxieties can occur in adulthood as well. This duration criterion helps to minimize over-diagnosis of transient social anxiety.

Criteria G, H, I, and J

Most individuals experience some social anxiety at some point in their lives. Criterion G requires that the symptoms cause considerable impairment or distress. This criterion prevents the overdiagnosis of social anxiety disorder.

Many disorders are characterized by fear of social situations. Social anxiety disorder should be diagnosed only when the avoidance is not attributable to the effects of a substance or medication, is not better explained by another mental disorder, and is not related to another medical condition (Criteria H, I, and I).

Specifiers

Evidence suggests that the "performance only" specifier represents a subset of the larger social anxiety disorder group with different pathophysiological correlates and treatment response.

Panic Disorder

Panic disorder is characterized by a pattern of recurrent panic attacks accompanied by persistent worry or behavioral change. Therefore, individuals with panic disorder experience anxiety symptoms and functional impairment independent of the actual attack. The panic attacks occur spontaneously, arising without any trigger or environmental cue. There has been considerable interest in the relationship between panic disorder and agoraphobia. Although DSM-IV described panic disorder both with agoraphobia and without agoraphobia, this distinction is not included in DSM-5 because it was not meaningful. Panic disorder often co-occurs with a number of mental conditions beyond agoraphobia, particularly anxiety and depressive disorders.

Panic disorder was included in DSM-III and was recognized as a distinct entity. From DSM-III through DSM-IV-TR, panic disorder and agoraphobia were tightly linked. As conceptualized in DSM-IV, agoraphobia invariably involves at least some form of spontaneous crescendo anxiety, even if such episodes do not meet formal criteria for panic attacks. In the earlier versions of DSM and in ICD-10, agoraphobia is considered less closely linked to panic disorder.

Diagnostic Criteria for Panic Disorder   **300.01** (F41.0)

A. Recurrent unexpected panic attacks. A panic attack is an abrupt surge of intense fear or intense discomfort that reaches a peak within minutes, and during which time four (or more) of the following symptoms occur:

Note: The abrupt surge can occur from a calm state or an anxious state.

1. Palpitations, pounding heart, or accelerated heart rate.
2. Sweating.
3. Trembling or shaking.
4. Sensations of shortness of breath or smothering.
5. Feelings of choking.
6. Chest pain or discomfort.
7. Nausea or abdominal distress.
8. Feeling dizzy, unsteady, light-headed, or faint.
9. Chills or heat sensations.
10. Paresthesias (numbness or tingling sensations).
11. Derealization (feelings of unreality) or depersonalization (being detached from oneself).
12. Fear of losing control or "going crazy."
13. Fear of dying.

Note: Culture-specific symptoms (e.g., tinnitus, neck soreness, headache, uncontrollable screaming or crying) may be seen. Such symptoms should not count as one of the four required symptoms.

B. At least one of the attacks has been followed by 1 month (or more) of one or both of the following:

1. Persistent concern or worry about additional panic attacks or their consequences (e.g., losing control, having a heart attack, "going crazy").
2. A significant maladaptive change in behavior related to the attacks (e.g., behaviors designed to avoid having panic attacks, such as avoidance of exercise or unfamiliar situations).

C. The disturbance is not attributable to the physiological effects of a substance (e.g., a drug of abuse, a medication) or another medical condition (e.g., hyperthyroidism, cardiopulmonary disorders).

D. The disturbance is not better explained by another mental disorder (e.g., the panic attacks do not occur only in response to feared social situations, as in social anxiety disorder; in response to circumscribed phobic objects or situations, as in specific phobia; in response to obsessions, as in obsessive-compulsive disorder; in response to reminders of traumatic events, as in posttraumatic stress disorder; or in response to separation from attachment figures, as in separation anxiety disorder).

Criteria A and B

Panic disorder requires recurrent and "unexpected" panic attacks, at least one of which is associated with either persistent concern or worry about additional attacks, or changes in behavior related to the attacks. Examples are provided to help the clinician understand the functional impact of the attacks.

Criteria C and D

Panic disorder must be differentiated from medical conditions that produce similar symptoms. Panic attacks have been associated with a variety of endocrinological disorders, including both hypo- and hyperthyroid states, hyperparathyroidism, and pheochromocytomas. Episodic hypoglycemia can also produce panic symptoms. Seizure disorders, vestibular dysfunction, neoplasms, prescribed and illicit substances, and cardiac and pulmonary problems (e.g., arrhythmias, chronic obstructive pulmonary disease, asthma) can all result in panic symptoms. Clues to an underlying medical cause for panic symptoms include atypical features during panic attacks, such as ataxia, alterations in consciousness, or bladder dyscontrol; onset of panic disorder relatively late in life; or physical signs and symptoms indicating a medical condition.

Panic disorder also must be differentiated from a number of mental disorders, particularly other anxiety states. Differentiation from generalized anxiety disorder can sometimes be difficult, but classic panic attacks are characterized by rapid onset and short duration, in contrast to the anxiety associated with generalized anxiety disorder, which emerges and dissipates more slowly. Anxiety also frequently accompanies many other psychiatric disorders, including psychotic and mood disorders.

Panic Attack Specifier

A panic attack is a sudden episode of intense fear or discomfort lasting minutes to hours that triggers uncomfortable physical sensations. Panic attacks usually begin abruptly, peak within minutes, and can be frightening to the individual. When they occur, the person may believe he or she is losing control, having a heart attack, or even dying. Although many people have isolated panic attacks during stressful times, these attacks do not occur repeatedly. Panic attacks may occur in various psychopathological states.

Freud's description of anxiety neurosis was defined by the coexistence of a state of moderate and permanent anxiety and of anxiety attacks, whose manifestations were similar to today's panic attack. Anxiety neurosis was later subdivided into the acute anxiety attack (i.e., a panic attack) and a state of moderate and continuous anxiety (now referred to as generalized anxiety disorder). This distinction was included in the Research Diagnostic Criteria (Spitzer et al. 1975) and appeared a few years later in DSM-III.

Importantly, as stated in DSM-5, panic attacks can be noted as a specifier for any anxiety disorder as well as for other mental disorders (e.g., depressive disorders, posttraumatic stress disorder) and some medical conditions (e.g., cardiac, respiratory, vestibular, gastrointestinal). When the presence of a panic attack is identified, it should be documented with the specifier "with panic attacks" (e.g., posttraumatic stress disorder with panic attacks).

Panic Attack Specifier

Note: Symptoms are presented for the purpose of identifying a panic attack; however, panic attack is not a mental disorder and cannot be coded. Panic attacks can occur in the context of any anxiety disorder as well as other mental disorders (e.g., depressive disorders, posttraumatic stress disorder, substance use disorders) and some medical conditions (e.g., cardiac, respiratory, vestibular, gastrointestinal). When the presence of a panic attack is identified, it should be noted as a specifier (e.g., "posttraumatic stress disorder with panic attacks"). For panic disorder, the presence of panic attack is contained within the criteria for the disorder and panic attack is not used as a specifier.

An abrupt surge of intense fear or intense discomfort that reaches a peak within minutes, and during which time four (or more) of the following symptoms occur:

Note: The abrupt surge can occur from a calm state or an anxious state.

1. Palpitations, pounding heart, or accelerated heart rate.
2. Sweating.
3. Trembling or shaking.
4. Sensations of shortness of breath or smothering.
5. Feelings of choking.
6. Chest pain or discomfort.
7. Nausea or abdominal distress.
8. Feeling dizzy, unsteady, light-headed, or faint.
9. Chills or heat sensations.
10. Paresthesias (numbness or tingling sensations).
11. Derealization (feelings of unreality) or depersonalization (being detached from oneself).
12. Fear of losing control or "going crazy."
13. Fear of dying.

Note: Culture-specific symptoms (e.g., tinnitus, neck soreness, headache, uncontrollable screaming or crying) may be seen. Such symptoms should not count as one of the four required symptoms.

By itself, a panic attack is not a codable disorder. Episodes of abrupt fear occur in many situations. A healthy person might experience a panic attack when confronted with sudden extreme danger, and an individual with a phobia of heights might experience a panic attack when confronted with the feared situation. DSM-5 requires that panic attacks be listed as a specifier to the specific disorder with which they occur. The importance of the specifier is based on data demonstrating that panic attacks predict the severity of other forms of psychopathology. A person who meets at least four of the symptoms qualifies as having a panic attack. Data from the DSM-IV field trial confirmed that the four-symptom threshold is optimal.

Although the DSM-5 symptoms are unchanged from DSM-IV, they are now rank-ordered from most to least common. In addition, "heat sensations" replaces the DSM-IV symptom "hot flushes." The concluding note is included to increase clinician awareness of culture-based symptoms. For example, higher rates of paresthesias occur in African Americans, trembling in Caribbean Latinos, and depersonalization/derealization in Puerto Ricans.

Agoraphobia

Agoraphobia was first identified by Westphal in the late 19th century when he described people who feared public places (Goodwin and Guze 1989). DSM-III introduced and codified agoraphobia as a distinctive syndrome characterized by "marked fear and avoidance of being alone or in public places from which escape might be difficult or help not available in case of sudden incapacitations" (p. 226). In DSM-III-R, agoraphobia was specifically defined as a classically conditioned response to panic attacks. Although agoraphobia could be diagnosed in the absence of a history of panic attacks, such an occurrence was thought to be rare. Therefore, agoraphobia became conceptually linked to panic attacks, but was also seen explicitly and exclusively as a secondary complication. In DSM-IV, agoraphobia could be diagnosed only within the context of panic disorder or as the result of panic attacks or panic-like symptoms (i.e., agoraphobia was related to fear of developing panic symptoms such as dizziness or diarrhea). In community samples, however, the majority of people with agoraphobia never experienced panic attacks or panic-like symptoms or psychophysiological symptoms of other types that clearly preceded the onset of agoraphobic avoidance. In DSM-5, agoraphobia is a codable disorder independent of panic disorder or panic attacks (Wittchen et al. 2010).

Diagnostic Criteria for Agoraphobia 300.22 (F40.00)

A. Marked fear or anxiety about two (or more) of the following five situations:
1. Using public transportation (e.g., automobiles, buses, trains, ships, planes).
2. Being in open spaces (e.g., parking lots, marketplaces, bridges).
3. Being in enclosed places (e.g., shops, theaters, cinemas).
4. Standing in line or being in a crowd.
5. Being outside of the home alone.

B. The individual fears or avoids these situations because of thoughts that escape might be difficult or help might not be available in the event of developing panic-like symptoms or other incapacitating or embarrassing symptoms (e.g., fear of falling in the elderly; fear of incontinence).

C. The agoraphobic situations almost always provoke fear or anxiety.

D. The agoraphobic situations are actively avoided, require the presence of a companion, or are endured with intense fear or anxiety.

E. The fear or anxiety is out of proportion to the actual danger posed by the agoraphobic situations and to the sociocultural context.

F. The fear, anxiety, or avoidance is persistent, typically lasting for 6 months or more.

G. The fear, anxiety, or avoidance causes clinically significant distress or impairment in social, occupational, or other important areas of functioning.

H. If another medical condition (e.g., inflammatory bowel disease, Parkinson's disease) is present, the fear, anxiety, or avoidance is clearly excessive.

I. The fear, anxiety, or avoidance is not better explained by the symptoms of another mental disorder—for example, the symptoms are not confined to specific phobia, situational type; do not involve only social situations (as in social anxiety disorder); and are not related exclusively to obsessions (as in obsessive-compulsive disorder), perceived defects or flaws in physical appearance (as in body dysmorphic disorder), reminders of traumatic events (as in posttraumatic stress disorder), or fear of separation (as in separation anxiety disorder).

Note: Agoraphobia is diagnosed irrespective of the presence of panic disorder. If an individual's presentation meets criteria for panic disorder and agoraphobia, both diagnoses should be assigned.

Criterion A

The person with agoraphobia must report fear or anxiety arising from at least two of the five general situations listed. The requirement of at least two such situations differentiates agoraphobia from a specific phobia, which may be limited to one particular situation. Also, the fear or anxiety is related exclusively to the situations and is not attributable to more generalized anxiety that the person experiences in multiple situations.

Criterion B

The diagnosis of agoraphobia requires the person to have a cognitive ideational component related to the fear or avoidance. This criterion emphasizes the motivation for the avoidance, such as fear that escape will be difficult. In addition, the cognitive aspect of agoraphobia can be associated with fear or avoidance of the situation because of thoughts that "help might not be available in the event of developing panic-like symptoms or other incapacitating or embarrassing symptoms (e.g., fear of falling in the elderly; fear of incontinence)," and thereby allows for the diagnosis in the absence of panic-like symptoms.

Criterion C

This criterion requires that the situations almost always provoke fear or anxiety and therefore raises the threshold for making the diagnosis. A single or even occasional event of avoiding situations due to fear would not qualify for the diagnosis.

Criterion D

DSM-5 includes the phrase "actively avoided" to minimize overdiagnosis of mild fears.

Criterion E

This criterion is new and is used to increase reliability and separation from normal fears. The criterion evokes clinician judgment (vs. self-recognition). For example, a person with a history of incontinence may refuse to leave home for long stretches of time, and that may be reasonable. If the person had only a single episode of incontinence and has refused to leave home for years, then that would be out of proportion to the fear.

Criterion F

To avoid overdiagnosis of transient fear or anxiety, the duration is indicated as typically for 6 months or more. This was previously not a requirement.

Criteria G, H, and I

The degree of impairment associated with agoraphobia can vary from only avoiding situations to being entirely housebound (Criterion G). This criterion is intended to increase separation of individuals with agoraphobia from those with mild or transient fears.

The core feature of agoraphobia is avoidance, a symptom that may be present in a number of other disorders. The clinician should rule out other medical conditions (e.g., inflammatory bowel disease) in which avoidance behavior may be present (Criterion H). Other mental disorders also need to be ruled out (e.g., obsessive-compulsive disorder) (Criterion I).

Generalized Anxiety Disorder

Generalized anxiety disorder is characterized by a pattern of frequent, persistent excessive anxiety and worry that is out of proportion to the impact of the event or circumstance that is the focus of the worry. Individuals with generalized anxiety disorder may not acknowledge the excessive nature of their worry, but they are bothered by their degree of worry. This pattern of worry occurs "more days than not for at least 6 months" (Criterion A). Individuals find it difficult to control this worry and report at least three of six somatic or cognitive symptoms (or one symptom for children).

Generalized anxiety disorder was first included in DSM-III, having been split off from anxiety neurosis. The disorder was originally considered a diagnosis of exclusion, because it could not be "attributable to another mental disorder." DSM-III also required a 1-month duration of symptoms, but concerns later arose about the low reliability of the diagnosis. In DSM-III-R, the duration was increased to 6 months and the symptom list was expanded. DSM-III-R also removed some of the hierarchical rules that had limited the diagnosis to individuals in whom the symptoms were not due to another disorder. Finally, in DSM-IV the list of associated symptoms was simplified from 18 to 6, of which individuals had to exhibit at least 3. More emphasis was placed on the pervasiveness of the worry, and the criteria were modified to accommodate childhood presentations. DSM-IV attempted to integrate the approach to worry across development. In DSM-5, the diagnosis is mostly unchanged from that in DSM-IV except for wording changes and a reorganization of the criteria.

Diagnostic Criteria for Generalized Anxiety Disorder   **300.02** (F41.1)

A. Excessive anxiety and worry (apprehensive expectation), occurring more days than not for at least 6 months, about a number of events or activities (such as work or school performance).

B. The individual finds it difficult to control the worry.

C. The anxiety and worry are associated with three (or more) of the following six symptoms (with at least some symptoms having been present for more days than not for the past 6 months):

Note: Only one item is required in children.

1. Restlessness or feeling keyed up or on edge.
2. Being easily fatigued.
3. Difficulty concentrating or mind going blank.
4. Irritability.
5. Muscle tension.
6. Sleep disturbance (difficulty falling or staying asleep, or restless, unsatisfying sleep).

D. The anxiety, worry, or physical symptoms cause clinically significant distress or impairment in social, occupational, or other important areas of functioning.
E. The disturbance is not attributable to the physiological effects of a substance (e.g., a drug of abuse, a medication) or another medical condition (e.g., hyperthyroidism).
F. The disturbance is not better explained by another mental disorder (e.g., anxiety or worry about having panic attacks in panic disorder, negative evaluation in social anxiety disorder [social phobia], contamination or other obsessions in obsessive-compulsive disorder, separation from attachment figures in separation anxiety disorder, reminders of traumatic events in posttraumatic stress disorder, gaining weight in anorexia nervosa, physical complaints in somatic symptom disorder, perceived appearance flaws in body dysmorphic disorder, having a serious illness in illness anxiety disorder, or the content of delusional beliefs in schizophrenia or delusional disorder).

Criteria A and B

Generalized anxiety disorder is not the same as normal worry, and these criteria are intended to distinguish the two. Worries considered sufficient for the disorder must be excessive. An evaluation of the intensity, frequency, and focus of worries provides clues to whether the anxiety is excessive. The minimum duration requirement of 6 months is set high enough to distinguish generalized anxiety disorder from episodic or short-lived events that cause worry. Furthermore, the person finds it difficult to control the worry.

Criterion C

This item includes both somatic and cognitive aspects of generalized anxiety disorder. The requirement of three or more symptoms for adults and one for children is unchanged from DSM-IV.

Criterion D

This criterion establishes a threshold by which normal worry will not become pathologized. The requirement that the worry cause significant distress or impairment should prevent an individual from receiving this diagnosis unless the worry is severe.

Criteria E and F

Anxiety is a frequent symptom of substance use and of several medical conditions, which must be ruled out. Anxiety or worry is also a defining or associated feature of many mental disorders. Criterion F provides examples of worries covered by other diagnoses and thereby reserves the diagnosis of generalized anxiety disorder to those worries not covered by other conditions. An additional diagnosis of generalized anxiety disorder, however, may be appropriate when the worries extend beyond the specific symptoms of another disorder.

Substance/Medication-Induced Anxiety Disorder

For individuals with a substance/medication-induced anxiety disorder, clinically significant symptoms of panic, worry, phobia, or obsessions emerge in the context of prescribed or illicit substance use. The differential diagnosis requires that substance use and medications be ruled out as possible causes of anxiety before one of the other anxiety disorders is diagnosed. Clinicians should routinely document the substance use status of all patients and record all medications.

Clinicians should be particularly attuned to substance misuse when encountering an anxious individual. If misuse is present, the clinician must then determine whether it has any relationship to the ongoing anxiety symptoms. Although no definitive test exists to establish such a causal relationship, several factors can help confirm the diagnosis. These include the timing of the symptoms, the existing literature pertaining to the strength of the association between anxiety and the potential complicating factor, and signs or symptoms that are atypical of an anxiety disorder.

Onset of anxiety symptoms may occur during substance intoxication or withdrawal, and onset of such symptoms is indicated by use of specifiers. Anxiety is associated with multiple illicit substances (e.g., amphetamines, cocaine), alcohol, and caffeine. The diagnosis can also be made when the anxiety is associated with use of prescription drugs (e.g., anticholinergics, antidepressants, lithium). A diagnosis of substance-induced anxiety disorder rather than substance intoxication or withdrawal is appropriate when the anxiety symptoms predominate and are in excess of what is expected and warrant independent clinical attention.

Diagnostic Criteria for Substance/Medication-Induced Anxiety Disorder

A. Panic attacks or anxiety is predominant in the clinical picture.
B. There is evidence from the history, physical examination, or laboratory findings of both (1) and (2):
   1. The symptoms in Criterion A developed during or soon after substance intoxication or withdrawal or after exposure to a medication.
   2. The involved substance/medication is capable of producing the symptoms in Criterion A.
C. The disturbance is not better explained by an anxiety disorder that is not substance/medication-induced. Such evidence of an independent anxiety disorder could include the following:

   The symptoms precede the onset of the substance/medication use; the symptoms persist for a substantial period of time (e.g., about 1 month) after the cessation of acute withdrawal or severe intoxication; or there is other evidence suggesting the existence of an independent non-substance/medication-induced anxiety disorder (e.g., a history of recurrent non-substance/medication-related episodes).

D. The disturbance does not occur exclusively during the course of a delirium.

E. The disturbance causes clinically significant distress or impairment in social, occupational, or other important areas of functioning.

Note: This diagnosis should be made instead of a diagnosis of substance intoxication or substance withdrawal only when the symptoms in Criterion A predominate in the clinical picture and they are sufficiently severe to warrant clinical attention.

Coding note: The ICD-9-CM and ICD-10-CM codes for the [specific substance/medication]-induced anxiety disorders are indicated in the table below. Note that the ICD-10-CM code depends on whether or not there is a comorbid substance use disorder present for the same class of substance. If a mild substance use disorder is comorbid with the substance-induced anxiety disorder, the 4th position character is "1," and the clinician should record "mild [substance] use disorder" before the substance-induced anxiety disorder (e.g., "mild cocaine use disorder with cocaine-induced anxiety disorder"). If a moderate or severe substance use disorder is comorbid with the substance-induced anxiety disorder, the 4th position character is "2," and the clinician should record "moderate [substance] use disorder" or "severe [substance] use disorder," depending on the severity of the comorbid substance use disorder. If there is no comorbid substance use disorder (e.g., after a one-time heavy use of the substance), then the 4th position character is "9," and the clinician should record only the substance-induced anxiety disorder.

		ICD-10-CM		
	ICD-9-CM	With use disorder, mild	With use disorder, moderate or severe	Without use disorder
Alcohol	291.89	F10.180	F10.280	F10.980
Caffeine	292.89	F15.180	F15.280	F15.980
Cannabis	292.89	F12.180	F12.280	F12.980
Phencyclidine	292.89	F16.180	F16.280	F16.980
Other hallucinogen	292.89	F16.180	F16.280	F16.980
Inhalant	292.89	F18.180	F18.280	F18.980
Opioid	292.89	F11.188	F11.288	F11.988
Sedative, hypnotic, or anxiolytic	292.89	F13.180	F13.280	F13.980
Amphetamine (or other stimulant)	292.89	F15.180	F15.280	F15.980
Cocaine	292.89	F14.180	F14.280	F14.980
Other (or unknown) substance	292.89	F19.180	F19.280	F19.980

Specify if (see Table 1 in the chapter "Substance-Related and Addictive Disorders" [in DSM-5] for diagnoses associated with substance class):

With onset during intoxication: This specifier applies if criteria are met for intoxication with the substance and the symptoms develop during intoxication.

With onset during withdrawal: This specifier applies if criteria are met for withdrawal from the substance and the symptoms develop during, or shortly after, withdrawal.

With onset after medication use: Symptoms may appear either at initiation of medication or after a modification or change in use.

Anxiety Disorder Due to Another Medical Condition

Anxiety symptoms can develop in the context of identifiable medical syndromes. Endocrine conditions (e.g., hyperthyroidism, hypoglycemia), cardiovascular conditions (e.g., arrhythmia, congestive heart failure), respiratory diseases (e.g., chronic obstructive pulmonary disease, pneumonia), neurological conditions (e.g., neoplasms, encephalitis), and metabolic conditions (e.g., vitamin B_{12} deficiency) all may be associated with anxiety. If another medical condition is present and determined to be the direct physiological cause of the anxiety symptoms, then anxiety disorder due to another medical condition should be diagnosed. When recording the diagnosis, the clinician should include the name of the other medical condition within the name of the mental disorder (e.g., 293.84 [F06.4] anxiety disorder due to pheochromocytoma). The other medical condition should be coded and listed separately immediately before the anxiety disorder due to the medical condition (e.g., 227.0 [D35.00] pheochromocytoma; 293.84 [F06.4] anxiety disorder due to pheochromocytoma).

Diagnostic Criteria for Anxiety Disorder Due to Another Medical Condition   **293.84** (F06.4)

A. Panic attacks or anxiety is predominant in the clinical picture.
B. There is evidence from the history, physical examination, or laboratory findings that the disturbance is the direct pathophysiological consequence of another medical condition.
C. The disturbance is not better explained by another mental disorder.
D. The disturbance does not occur exclusively during the course of a delirium.
E. The disturbance causes clinically significant distress or impairment in social, occupational, or other important areas of functioning.

Coding note: Include the name of the other medical condition within the name of the mental disorder (e.g., 293.84 [F06.4] anxiety disorder due to pheochromocytoma). The other medical condition should be coded and listed separately immediately before the anxiety disorder due to the medical condition (e.g., 227.0 [D35.00] pheochromocytoma; 293.84 [F06.4] anxiety disorder due to pheochromocytoma.

Other Specified Anxiety Disorder and Unspecified Anxiety Disorder

Because anxiety represents one of the most common psychiatric symptoms, it is not uncommon to encounter individuals who have impairment from anxiety but whose symptoms do not meet criteria for one of the specific anxiety disorders. These individuals are appropriately classified as having an other specified or unspecified anxiety disorder.

The categories replace DSM-IV's anxiety disorder not otherwise specified. Other specified anxiety disorder is used when symptoms characteristic of an anxiety disorder are present and cause distress or impairment but do not meet the full criteria for a more specific disorder in the class. The category is used when the clinician chooses to communicate the reason that the presentation does not meet full criteria. The clinician is encouraged to record the specific reason (e.g., limited-symptom attacks).

The category unspecified anxiety disorder is used when the individual's symptoms do not meet full criteria for a more specific disorder that causes distress or impairment, and the clinician chooses not to specify the reason the criteria are not met or there is insufficient information to make a more specific diagnosis.

Other Specified Anxiety Disorder   **300.09** (F41.8)

This category applies to presentations in which symptoms characteristic of an anxiety disorder that cause clinically significant distress or impairment in social, occupational, or other important areas of functioning predominate but do not meet the full criteria for any of the disorders in the anxiety disorders diagnostic class. The other specified anxiety disorder category is used in situations in which the clinician chooses to communicate the specific reason that the presentation does not meet the criteria for any specific anxiety disorder. This is done by recording "other specified anxiety disorder" followed by the specific reason (e.g., "generalized anxiety not occurring more days than not").

Examples of presentations that can be specified using the "other specified" designation include the following:

1. **Limited-symptom attacks.**
2. **Generalized anxiety not occurring more days than not.**
3. ***Khyâl cap* (wind attacks):** See "Glossary of Cultural Concepts of Distress" in the Appendix to DSM-5.
4. ***Ataque de nervios* (attack of nerves):** See "Glossary of Cultural Concepts of Distress" in the Appendix to DSM-5.

Unspecified Anxiety Disorder   **300.00** (F41.9)

This category applies to presentations in which symptoms characteristic of an anxiety disorder that cause clinically significant distress or impairment in social, occupational, or other important areas of functioning predominate but do not meet the full criteria for any of the disorders in the anxiety disorders diagnostic class. The unspecified anxiety disorder category is used in situations in which the clinician chooses *not* to specify the reason that the criteria are not met for a specific anxiety disorder, and includes presentations in which there is insufficient information to make a more specific diagnosis (e.g., in emergency room settings).

KEY POINTS

- The anxiety disorders class no longer includes obsessive-compulsive disorder, posttraumatic stress disorder, or acute stress disorder. Separation anxiety disorder and selective mutism have been added to the class. The wording of the former has been changed to more adequately represent the expression of separation anxiety symptoms in adulthood.

- For specific phobia and social anxiety disorder, changes to the criteria include deletion of the requirement that adults recognize their anxiety as excessive or unreasonable. Instead, the anxiety should be "out of proportion" to the actual danger or threat, after sociocultural factors are taken into account. The typical minimum 6-month duration, which was limited to individuals younger than age 18 years, has been extended to persons of all ages.

- The specific phobia criteria are reworded so that the chance of encountering the phobic stimulus is no longer a determinant of whether an individual receives the diagnosis. The different stimulus types of specific phobias (now specifiers) are mostly unchanged.

- With social anxiety disorder, the "generalized" specifier has been dropped and replaced with a "performance only" specifier.

- Panic disorder and agoraphobia have been unlinked. The specifier "with panic attacks" can be used for any anxiety disorder, other mental disorders, and some medical conditions.

References

Goodwin D, Guze S: Psychiatric Diagnosis, 4th Edition. New York, Oxford University Press, 1989

Spitzer RL, Endicott J, Robins E: Research diagnostic criteria (RDC). New York, Biometrics Research, New York State Psychiatric Institute, 1975

Wittchen HU, Gloster AT, Beesdo-Baum K, et al: Agoraphobia: a review of the diagnostic classificatory position and criteria. Depress Anxiety 27:113–133, 2010

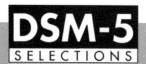

Anxiety Disorders

DSM-5® Clinical Cases

Introduction

John W. Barnhill, M.D.

The DSM-5 chapter on anxiety disorders brings together a cluster of presentations in which anxiety, fear, and avoidance are prominent. Among the most prevalent psychiatric diagnoses, anxiety disorders can also be among the most difficult to definitively diagnose. One complicating factor is that anxiety, fear, and avoidance are normal and adaptive responses, leading to some inevitable ambiguity in evaluations of people with mild symptoms.

Another factor is that anxiety-related emotions can be most prominently experienced as somatic symptoms. Fear—a normal response to a real or perceived imminent threat—is almost always associated with autonomic hyperarousal; such hyperarousal can be difficult for patients to identify or describe, especially if it is chronic. Similarly, anxiety—the emotional experience of fear unaccompanied by a clear threat—may be experienced as muscle tension and vigilance, which can blend imperceptibly into background noise for someone with chronically elevated anxiety levels.

A third complication is that anxiety disorders are often comorbid with one another and with mood and personality disorders, which can make it difficult to adequately attend to the manifestations of each diagnosis.

Finally, definitions of anxiety disorders are descriptive of phenomena with unknown pathophysiologies, and despite many advances, the field of psychiatry is not yet close to definitively identifying nosological categories based on underlying etiology.

One important diagnostic shift involves panic, which is described in two different ways in DSM-5. Panic attacks are now understood to occur as part of a broad spectrum of psychiatric diagnoses and to have significance in regard to severity, course, and morbidity, and they can now be identified as a specifier for all DSM-5 anxiety disorders, as well as for some other DSM-5 disorders. Panic attacks can be subtyped simply as expected or unexpected. When persistent panic attacks induce an ongoing, significant fear of further panic attacks, panic disorder is the likely diagnosis.

Historically linked to panic disorder, agoraphobia is identified in DSM-5 as a distinct diagnosis that can develop in the context of a variety of stressors and psychiatric syndromes. As with specific phobia and social anxiety disorder, agoraphobia no longer requires that individuals over age 18 perceive the anxiety as unreasonable. Instead, the clinician can make a judgment as to whether the anxiety is out of proportion to the actual danger or threat. To reduce the likelihood of overdiagnosing transient fears, these disorders must persist for at least 6 months for all individuals rather than just for those under age 18.

A significant structural shift within DSM-5 is the movement of separation anxiety disorder into the chapter on anxiety disorders. Separation anxiety disorder still requires an onset before age 18, but the hope is that with a general adult population prevalence of over 6%, it will be more commonly addressed in adults than it has been in the past, when the disorder was listed among disorders of children and adolescents.

Another significant structural change among the DSM-5 anxiety-related disorders is the shift of obsessive-compulsive disorder and posttraumatic stress disorder into their own chapters. These new chapters include clusters of disorders in which anxiety plays a prominent role but which also have other features (e.g., obsessions/compulsions or a significant trauma history).

The various anxiety-related disorders can often be clearly differentiated, but they can also be difficult to distinguish and can often be comorbid with each other and with most other psychiatric diagnoses. A chief complaint of "anxiety" does not make the diagnosis but is instead the beginning of a clinical thought process that can range throughout DSM-5.

Suggested Readings

Horwitz AV, Wakefield JC: All We Have to Fear: Psychiatry's Transformation of Natural Anxieties Into Mental Disorders. New York, Oxford University Press, 2012

Milrod B: The Gordian knot of clinical research in anxiety disorders: some answers, more questions. Am J Psychiatry 170(7):703–706, 2013

Stein DJ, Hollander E, Rothbaum BO (eds): Textbook of Anxiety Disorders, 2nd Edition. Washington, DC, American Psychiatric Publishing, 2010

Case 1: Fears and Worries

Loes Jongerden, M.A.
Susan Bögels, Ph.D.

Logan was a 12-year-old boy who was referred to mental health care for long-standing anxiety about losing his parents and relatively recent fears about getting a severe disease.

Although his parents described a long history of anxiety, Logan's acute problem began 5 weeks prior to the consultation, when he watched a television show about rare and fatal diseases. Afterward, he became scared that he might have a hidden disease. His parents reported three "panic attacks" in the prior month, marked by anxiety, dizziness, sweats, and shortness of breath. About that same time, Logan began to complain of frequent headaches and stomachaches. Logan's own theory was that his bodily aches were caused by his fears about being ill and about his parents going away, but the pain was still uncomfortable. He insisted he was not scared about having more panic attacks but was petrified about being left sick and alone. These illness fears developed several times a week, usually when Logan was in bed, when he "felt something" in his body, or when he heard about diseases.

Logan had begun to suffer from anxieties as a young child. Kindergarten was notable for intense separation difficulties. He was briefly bullied in third grade, which led to his first panic attacks and worsening anxiety. According to his parents, "there always seemed to be a new anxiety." These included fear of the toilet, the dark, sleeping alone, being alone, and being pestered.

Logan's most persistent fear revolved around his parents' safety. He was generally fine when both were at work or at home, but when they were in transit, or anywhere else, he was generally afraid that they would die in an accident. When the parents were late from work or when they tried to go out together or on an errand without him, Logan became frantic, calling and texting incessantly. Logan was predominantly concerned about his mother's safety, and she had gradually reduced her solo activities to a minimum. As she said, it felt like "he would like to follow me into the toilet." Logan was less demanding toward his father, who said, "When we comfort him all the time or stay at home, he'll never become independent." He indicated that he believed his wife had been too soft and overprotective.

Logan and his family underwent several months of psychotherapy when Logan was age 10. The father said therapy helped his wife become less overprotective, and Logan's anxiety seemed to improve. She agreed with this assessment, although she said she was not sure what she was supposed to do when her son was panicking whenever she tried to leave the house or whenever he worried about getting a disease.

Logan's developmental history was otherwise unremarkable. His grades were generally good. His teachers agreed that he was quiet but had several friends and collaborated well with other children. He was quick, however, to negatively interpret the intentions of other children. For example, he tended to be very sensitive to any indication that he was being picked on.

Logan's family history was pertinent for panic disorder, agoraphobia, and social anxiety disorder (social phobia) in the mother. The maternal grandmother was described as "at least as" anxious as Logan's mother. The father denied psychiatric illness in his family.

On examination, Logan was a friendly, articulate boy who was cooperative and goal directed. He was generally in a "good mood" but cried when talking about his fears of dying and getting sick. He denied suicidality and hopelessness but indicated he was desperate to get over his problems before starting high school. His cognition was good. His insight and judgment appeared intact except as related to his anxiety issues.

Diagnosis

• Separation anxiety disorder with panic attacks

Discussion

Logan has had separation fears since he was a young child. To qualify for separation anxiety disorder, DSM-5 requires three of eight symptoms. Logan has at least five, including long-standing, excessive, and disturbing fears of anticipated separations; of harm to his parents; of events that could lead to separations; and of being left alone. He also had physical complaints that could be traced to fears of dying and separation.

Logan also has panic attacks. He does not meet criteria for a panic disorder, however, because he is not afraid of having an attack. Instead, his panic seems related to fears of separation or getting a disease. Panic attacks would, therefore, be listed as a specifier of separation anxiety disorder.

Although Logan is anxious about having an illness, his symptoms do not appear to meet criteria for illness anxiety disorder: the duration of his fear of diseases is not 6 months, he does not visit doctors, and he seeks reassurance not about his health but about being left alone by his attachment figures. His symptoms do not meet criteria for generalized anxiety disorder because his predominant concern is specifically about separation from his parents. He may have met criteria for social anxiety disorder (social phobia) in the past (fear of being pestered), but social fears do not appear to dominate the clinical picture at this point in time.

Anxiety disorders have been present in the mother and grandmother, which may indicate a genetic predisposition. Multigenerational anxiety may also be transmitted via learning, modeling, and overprotective parenting. In Logan's case, the mother is noted to have panic disorder, agoraphobia, and social anxiety disorder, and both parents agree that her own anxieties have influenced her parenting style. In particular, Logan's fears appear to be rewarded: the parents stay home, rarely leave Logan alone, and respond quickly to all his calls and text messages. They appear to have frequent conversations about his fears but may not spend enough time discussing compensatory strategies. The father does seem to try to encourage Logan's autonomy, but the parents appear to not agree on the correct overall strategy. Unsupportive coparenting may have contributed to the maintenance of Logan's problems.

One potentially important change in DSM-5 has been the relocation of separation anxiety disorder into the anxiety disorder chapter. In DSM-III and DSM-IV, it was located in the chapter aimed at disorders that begin in infancy, childhood, and adolescence. Separation anxiety disorder can extend into adulthood, however, and Logan's mother may herself have suffered from adult separation anxiety disorder (as well as from her other anxiety disorders). Her own fears of separation may well be affecting how she is raising her son and be contributing to his ongoing anxiety.

Suggested Readings

Bögels S, Phares V: Fathers' role in the etiology, prevention and treatment of child anxiety: a review and new model. Clin Psychol Rev 28(4):539–558, 2008

Kessler RC, Berglund P, Demler O, et al: Lifetime prevalence and age-of-onset distributions of DSM-IV disorders in the National Comorbidity Survey Replication. Arch Gen Psychiatry 62(6):593–602, 2005

Majdandzic M, de Vente W, Feinberg ME, et al: Bidirectional associations between coparenting relations and family member anxiety: a review and conceptual model. Clin Child Fam Psychol Rev 15(1):28–42, 2012

McLeod BD, Wood JJ, Weisz JR: Examining the association between parenting and childhood anxiety: a meta-analysis. Clin Psychol Rev 27(2):155–172, 2007

van der Bruggen CO, Stams GJM, Bögels SM: Research review: the relation between child and parent anxiety and parental control: a meta-analytic review. J Child Psychol Psychiatry 49(12):1257–1269, 2008

Case 2: Panic

Carlo Faravelli, M.D.

Maria Greco was a 23-year-old single woman who was referred for psychiatric evaluation by her cardiologist. In the prior 2 months, she had presented to the emergency room four times for acute complaints of palpitations, shortness of breath, sweats, trembling, and the fear that she was about to die. Each of these events had a rapid onset. The symptoms peaked within minutes, leaving her scared, exhausted, and fully convinced that she had just experienced a heart attack. Medical evaluations done right after these episodes yielded normal physical exam findings, vital signs, lab results, toxicology screens, and electrocardiograms.

The patient reported a total of five such attacks in the prior 3 months, with the panic occurring at work, at home, and while driving a car. She had developed a persistent fear of having other attacks, which led her to take many days off work and to avoid exercise, driving, and coffee. Her sleep quality declined, as did her mood. She avoided social relationships. She did not accept the reassurance offered to her by friends and physicians, believing that the medical workups were negative because they were performed after the resolution of the symptoms. She continued to suspect that something was wrong with her heart and that without an accurate diagnosis, she was going to die. When she had a panic attack while asleep in the middle of the night, she finally agreed to see a psychiatrist.

Ms. Greco denied a history of previous psychiatric disorders except for a history of anxiety during childhood that had been diagnosed as a "school phobia."

The patient's mother had committed suicide by overdose 4 years earlier in the context of a recurrent major depression. At the time of the evaluation, the patient was living with her father and two younger siblings. The patient had graduated from high school, was working as a telephone operator, and was not dating anyone. Her family and social histories were otherwise noncontributory.

On examination, the patient was an anxious-appearing, cooperative, coherent young woman. She denied depression but did appear worried and was preoccupied with ideas of having heart disease. She denied psychotic symptoms, confusion, and all suicidality. Her cognition was intact, insight was limited, and judgment was fair.

Diagnosis

- Panic disorder

Discussion

Ms. Greco has panic attacks, which are abrupt surges of fear and/or discomfort that peak within minutes and are accompanied by physical and/or cognitive symptoms. In DSM-5, panic attacks are seen as a particular kind of fear response and are not found only in anxiety disorders. As such, panic is conceptualized in two ways within DSM-5. The first is as a "panic attack" specifier that can accompany any DSM-5 diagnosis. The second is as a panic disorder when the individual meets the more restrictive criteria for the disorder.

Ms. Greco appears to satisfy the multiple criteria required for panic disorder. First, her panic attacks are recurrent, and she more than meets the requirement for four of 13 panic symptoms: palpitations, sweating, trembling, smothering, chest pain, and a persistent fear of dying. The diagnosis also requires that the panic attacks affect the person between episodes. Not only does she constantly worry about having a heart attack (despite medical workups and frequent reassurance), she avoids situations and activities that might trigger another panic attack. These symptoms also have to last at least 1 month (Ms. Greco has been symptomatic for 2 months).

The diagnosis of panic disorder also requires an evaluation for the many other causes of panic. These include medications, medical illness, substances of abuse, and other mental disorders. According to the history, this 23-year-old woman takes no medications, has no medical illness, and denies use of substances of abuse. Her physical examinations, electrocardiograms, routine lab results, and toxicology screens are either normal or negative. It might be useful to ask Ms. Greco specifically about herbal and complementary medications, but it appears that her symptoms are psychiatric in origin.

Many psychiatric disorders are associated with panic, and Ms. Greco may have been primed for panic attacks by another condition. She reports a childhood history of anxiety and "social phobia," although those symptoms appear to have remitted. Her mother killed herself 4 years earlier in the context of a recurrent major depression. Details are unknown. Such a traumatic event would undoubtedly have some sort of effect on Ms. Greco. In fact, there would likely be two different traumas: the abrupt effects of the suicide and the more long-standing effects of having a chronically or recurrently depressed mother. Further exploration might focus on the psychosocial events leading up to these panic attacks.

For example, Ms. Greco's "school phobia" may have been a manifestation of undiagnosed separation anxiety disorder, and her recent panic may have developed in the setting of dating, sexual exploration, and/or a move away from her father and younger siblings. She does not present a pattern of panic in response to social anxiety or a specific phobia, but she also denies that her symptoms are psychiatric, and so may not recognize the link between her panic symptoms and another set of symptoms. It might be useful to assess Ms. Greco for anxiety sensitivity, which is the tendency to view anxiety as harmful, and for "negative affectivity," which is the proneness to experience negative emotions. Both of these personality traits may be associated with the development of panic.

Because certain symptom clusters are often not recognized spontaneously by patients as either symptoms or clusters of symptoms, it would be useful to look more specifically for such disorders as posttraumatic stress disorder and obsessive-compulsive disorder. In addition, it might be helpful to explore the sequence of symptoms. For example, the patient's panic seems to have led to her worries about heart disease. If the illness worries *preceded* the panic, she might also have an illness anxiety disorder or somatic symptom disorder.

Frequently comorbid with panic are depressive and bipolar disorders. Ms. Greco does have depressive symptoms, including insomnia and a preoccupation with death, but otherwise her symptoms do not appear to meet the criteria for a depression diagnosis. Her symptoms would, however, need to be observed longitudinally. Not only does her mother's history of depression increase her risk for depression, but she may not be especially insightful into her own emotional states. It would also be useful to specifically look for symptoms of bipolar disorder. Mania and hypomania are often forgotten by patients or are not perceived as problematic, and a missed diagnosis could lead to inappropriate treatment and an exacerbation of bipolar symptoms. Furthermore, the development of panic appears to increase the risk of suicide.

Although more should be explored, Ms. Greco does appear to have a panic disorder. DSM-5 suggests the assessment of whether the panic is expected or unexpected. It appears that Ms. Greco's initial panic attacks occurred in situations that might have been seen as stressful, such as while driving and at work, and so may or may not have been expected. Her last episode happened while she was asleep, however, so her panic attacks would be classified as unexpected.

DSM-5 has delinked agoraphobia from panic disorder. They can be comorbid, but agoraphobia is now recognized as developing in a variety of situations. In Ms. Greco's case, her active avoidance of driving, exercise, and caffeine is better conceptualized as a behavioral complication of panic disorder rather than a symptom of agoraphobia. Accurate diagnosis and treatment are important to prevent her symptoms from becoming more severe and chronic.

Suggested Readings

Faravelli C, Gorini Amedei S, Scarpato MA, et al: Bipolar disorder: an impossible diagnosis. Clin Pract Epidemiol Ment Health 5:13, 2009

Goodwin RD, Lieb R, Hoefler M, et al: Panic attack as a risk factor for severe psychopathology. Am J Psychiatry 161(12): 2207–2214, 2004

MacKinnon DF, Zandi PP, Cooper J, et al: Comorbid bipolar disorder and panic disorder in families with a high prevalence of bipolar disorder. Am J Psychiatry 159(1):30–35, 2002

Case 3: Adolescent Shyness

Barbara L. Milrod, M.D.

Nadine was a 15-year-old girl whose mother brought her for a psychiatric evaluation to help with her long-standing shyness.

Although Nadine was initially reluctant to say much about herself, she said she felt constantly tense. She added that the anxiety had been "really bad" for several years and was often accompanied by episodes of dizziness and crying. She was generally unable to speak in any situation outside of her home or school classes. She refused to leave her house alone for fear of being forced to interact with someone. She was especially anxious around other teenagers, but she had also become "too nervous" to speak to adult neighbors she had known for years. She said it felt impossible to walk into a restaurant and order from "a stranger at the counter" for fear of being humiliated. She also felt constantly on her guard, needing to avoid the possibility of getting attacked, a strategy that really only worked when she was alone in her home.

Nadine tried to conceal her crippling anxiety from her parents, typically telling them that she "just didn't feel like" going out. Feeling trapped and incompetent, Nadine said she contemplated suicide "all the time."

Nadine had always been "shy" and had been teased at recess since she started kindergarten. The teasing had escalated to outright bullying by the time she was in seventh grade. For two years, day after difficult day, Nadine's peers turned on her "like a snarling wolf pack," calling her "stupid," "ugly," and "crazy." Not infrequently, one of them would stare at her and tell her she would be better off committing suicide. One girl (the ringleader, as well as a former elementary school chum) hit Nadine on one occasion, giving her a black eye. Nadine did not fight back. This event was witnessed by an adult neighbor, who told Nadine's mother. When Nadine's mother asked her about the incident, Nadine denied it, saying she had "fallen" on the street. She did, however, mention to her mother "in passing" that she wanted to switch schools, but her delivery was so offhand that at the time, her mother casually advised against the switch. Nadine suffered on, sobbing herself to sleep most nights.

Full of hope, Nadine transferred to a specialty arts high school for ninth grade. Although the bullying ceased, her anxiety symptoms worsened. She felt even more unable to venture into public spaces and felt increasingly embarrassed by her inability to develop the sort of independence typical of a 15-year-old. She said she had begun to spend whole weekends "trapped" in her home and had become scared to even read by herself in the local park. She had nightly nightmares about the bullies in her old school. Her preoccupation with suicide grew.

Her parents had thought she would outgrow being shy and sought psychiatric help for her only after a teacher remarked that her anxiety and social isolation were keeping her from making the sort of grades and doing the sort of extracurricular activities that were necessary to get into a good college.

Nadine described her mother as loud, excitable, aggressive, and "a little frightening." Her father was a successful tax attorney who worked long hours. Nadine described him as shy in social situations ("He's more like me"). Nadine said she and her father sometimes joked that the goal of the evening was to avoid tipping the mother into a rage. Nadine added that she "never wanted to be anything like her mother."

Diagnoses

- Social anxiety disorder (social phobia), severe
- Posttraumatic stress disorder, moderate
- Agoraphobia, severe

Discussion

Nadine appears to have an underlying shy temperament. Unfortunately, with sandbox logic, shy children are often picked on. If they never learn adequate ways to defend themselves, bullying can escalate, particularly during their middle and high school years. This pattern can lead these anxiety-prone and already high-risk adolescents to be traumatized by their peers. As seen in Nadine, the intensity of the anxiety symptoms and the social isolation can combine to increase the risk of suicidal thoughts and behaviors.

By the time Nadine saw a psychiatrist, her distress had persisted for years and she appears to have developed a cluster of three DSM-5 diagnoses that are frequently comorbid. First, she has marked and excessive anxiety about multiple social situations, including ones with her peers. These situations always invoke fears of embarrassment, and are almost always avoided. She meets symptomatic criteria, therefore, for social anxiety disorder (social phobia).

As is common among children and adolescents, Nadine's fears took on a life of their own after the bullying experience. She initially avoided anxiety-provoking social situations, which is an aspect of her social anxiety disorder. That anxiety gradually expanded and exploded, however, and she began to panic if she tried to even leave her house by herself. When she became persistently unable to even go alone to a nearby park, she would be said to have a second DSM-5 diagnosis, agoraphobia. Such expansion is so common among children and adolescents that contemporary treatment studies tend to focus interventions on a range of DSM-defined anxiety disorders rather than on a single disorder.

Nadine should also be considered for a third DSM-5 diagnosis: posttraumatic stress disorder (PTSD). She has experienced intense and prolonged bullying, which is quite traumatic, especially when the child is socially isolated and going through a vulnerable period of development. To meet DSM-5 criteria for PTSD, Nadine would need to manifest clinically significant symptoms for at least 1 month in four different areas: intrusion (the nightmares, which she reported nightly), avoidance (of peers), negative alterations of cognitions and mood (exaggerated and negative views about herself), and alterations in arousal and reactivity (always on her guard). Because some of these symptoms can also refer to Nadine's social phobia, clinical judgment is required to avoid overdiagnosing PTSD. Nevertheless, it does appear that these two conditions are comorbid in Nadine. It is also important to explore the possibility that these anxiety symptoms might be attributable to a nonpsychiatric medical condition or to the use of medications or substances, but none of these appear to be involved in Nadine's case.

It is useful to recall, when evaluating the sort of adolescent trauma that Nadine experienced, that while other children are generally the bullies, teachers and administrators contribute to the problem by paying inadequate attention to schoolyard dynamics. This appears to be true in Nadine's case. In addition, Nadine's parents seem to have been able to ignore her desperate situation, until they became concerned about college admissions.

It is also useful to recognize that Nadine's mother is a loud, explosive woman whom Nadine has avoided "upsetting" since very early childhood. This tenuous mother-child relationship likely played a formative role in Nadine's shyness. Fear of her mother's explosions might have contributed to Nadine's persistent sense that she was not safe, for example, and might have prevented her from developing the tools that she needed to be successfully assertive. As the psychiatric evaluation evolves, it might be reasonable to discuss with Nadine the possibility that her failure to defend herself against the bullying might be related to her intense desire not to be anything like her loud and frightening mother.

Suggested Reading

Walkup JT, Albano AM, Piacentini J, et al: Cognitive behavioral therapy, sertraline, or a combination in childhood anxiety. N Engl J Med 359(26):2753–2766, 2008

Case 4: Flying Fears

Katharina Meyerbröker, Ph.D.

Olaf Hendricks, a 51-year-old businessman, presented to an outpatient psychiatrist complaining of his inability to travel by plane. His only daughter had just delivered a baby, and although he desperately wanted to meet his first granddaughter, he felt unable to fly across the Atlantic Ocean to where his daughter lived.

The patient's anxiety about flying had begun 3 years earlier when he was on a plane that landed in the middle of an ice storm. He had last flown 2 years earlier, reporting that he had cried on takeoff and landing. He had gone with his wife to an airport one additional time, 1 year prior to the evaluation, to fly to his daughter's wedding. Despite having drunk a significant amount of alcohol, Mr. Hendricks had panicked and refused to board the airplane. After that failed effort, he tended to feel intense anxiety when he even considered the possibility of flying, and the anxiety had led him to decline a promotion at work and an external job offer because both would have involved business trips.

Mr. Hendricks described sadness and regret since realizing his limitation but denied other neurovegetative symptoms of depression. He had increased his alcohol consumption to three glasses of wine nightly in order to "unwind." He denied any history of alcohol complications or withdrawal symptoms. He also denied a family history of psychiatric problems.

He denied anxiety in other situations, indicating that his colleagues saw him as a forceful and successful businessman who could "easily" deliver speeches in front of hundreds of people. When specifically asked, he reported that as a child, he had been "petrified" that he might get attacked by a wild animal. This fear had led him to refuse to go on family camping trips or even on long hikes in the country. As an adult, he said that he had no worries about being attacked by wild animals because he lived in a large city and took vacations by train to other large urban areas.

Diagnoses

- Specific phobia, situational (flying on airplanes)
- Specific phobia, animals

Discussion

Mr. Hendricks has such intense anxiety about flying that he will not get on airplanes despite being intensely motivated to do so. Even the thought of airplanes and airports causes significant distress. This fear is persistent and has caused significant functional impairment. He meets diagnostic criteria, therefore, for specific phobia. DSM-5 also includes specifiers to describe the phobia. In Mr. Hendricks's case, the phobic stimulus is flying, which would be coded as a "situational" specifier. (Other common situational stimuli include elevators and enclosed spaces.)

Most people with specific phobia fear more than one object or situation. Although Mr. Hendricks initially denies other anxieties, he does describe having had a highly distressing fear of being attacked by wild animals when he was younger. This fear led him to skip camping trips and hikes. He now lives in an urban environment where he is highly unlikely to come across a wild animal, but DSM-5 allows for a diagnosis of a specific phobia even when the phobic stimulus is not likely to be encountered. From a clinical perspective, uncovering such phobias is important because avoidance can not only cause fairly obvious distress and dysfunction (an inability to fly leading to an inability to visit family or optimally perform at work) but can also lead to life decisions that may not be completely conscious (a fear of wild animals leading to systematic avoidance of non-urban areas).

In addition to animals and situations, there are a number of other categories of phobic stimuli. These include the natural environment (e.g., heights, storms), blood-injection-injury (e.g., needles, invasive medical procedures), and other stimuli (e.g., loud sounds or costumed characters).

Specific phobia is most often comorbid with other anxiety disorders as well as depressive, substance use, somatic symptom, and personality disorders. Mr. Hendricks denies that his alcohol use is causing distress or dysfunction, so it does not appear to meet criteria for a DSM-5 disorder, but further exploration might indicate that his nightly drinking is causing problems with some aspect of his life. If it turns out that the flying phobia is a symptom of another disorder (e.g., one manifestation of agoraphobia), then the other disorder (the agoraphobia) would be the more accurate DSM-5 diagnosis. As it stands, however, Mr. Hendricks appears to have fairly classic specific phobia.

Suggested Readings

Emmelkamp PMG: Specific and social phobias in ICD-11. World Psychiatry 11(suppl 1):93–98, 2012

LeBeau RT, Glenn D, Liao B, et al: Specific phobia: a review of DSM-IV specific phobia and preliminary recommendations for DSM-V. Depress Anxiety 27(2):148–167, 2010

Zimmerman M, Dalrymple K, Chelminski I, et al: Recognition of irrationality of fear and the diagnosis of social anxiety disorder and specific phobia in adults: implications for criteria revision in DSM-5. Depress Anxiety 27(11):1044–1049, 2010

Case 5: Always on Edge

Ryan E. Lawrence, M.D.
Deborah L. Cabaniss, M.D.

Peggy Isaac was a 41-year-old administrative assistant who was referred for an outpatient evaluation by her primary care physician with a chief complaint of "I'm always on edge." She lived alone and had never married or had children. She had never before seen a psychiatrist.

Ms. Isaac had lived with her longtime boyfriend until 8 months earlier, at which time he had abruptly ended the relationship to date a younger woman. Soon thereafter, Ms. Isaac began to agonize about routine tasks and the possibility of making mistakes at work. She felt uncharacteristically tense and fatigued. She had difficulty focusing.

She also started to worry excessively about money and, to economize, she moved into a cheaper apartment in a less desirable neighborhood. She repeatedly sought reassurance from her office mates and her mother. No one seemed able to help, and she worried about being "too much of a burden."

During the 3 months prior to the evaluation, Ms. Isaac began to avoid going out at night, fearing that something bad would happen and she would be unable to summon help. More recently, she avoided going out in the daytime as well. She also felt "exposed and vulnerable" walking to the grocery store three blocks away, so she avoided shopping. After describing that she had figured out how to get her food delivered, she added, "It's ridiculous. I honestly feel something terrible is going to happen in one of the aisles and no one will help me, so I won't even go in." When in her apartment, she could often relax and enjoy a good book or movie.

Ms. Isaac said she had "always been a little nervous." Through much of kindergarten, she had cried inconsolably when her mother tried to drop her off. She reported seeing a counselor at age 10, during her parents' divorce, because "my mother thought I was too clingy." She added that she had never liked being alone, having had boyfriends constantly (occasionally overlapping) since age 16. She explained, "I hated being single, and I was always pretty, so I was never single for very long." Nevertheless, until the recent breakup, she said she had always thought of herself as "fine." She had been successful at work, jogged daily, maintained a solid network of friends, and had "no real complaints."

On initial interview, Ms. Isaac said she had been sad for a few weeks after her boyfriend left, but denied ever having felt worthless, guilty, hopeless, anhedonic, or suicidal. She said her weight was unchanged and her sleep was fine. She denied psychomotor changes. She did describe significant anxiety, with a Beck Anxiety Inventory score of 28, indicating severe anxiety.

Diagnosis

• Generalized anxiety disorder

Discussion

Ms. Isaac has become edgy, easily fatigued, and excessively worried during the 8 months since her boyfriend broke up with her. She has difficulty focusing. Her worries cause distress and dysfunction and lead her to repeatedly seek out reassurance. Although some of these symptoms could also be attributable to a depressive disorder, she lacks most other symptoms of a major depression. Instead, Ms. Isaac meets criteria for DSM-5 generalized anxiety disorder (GAD).

More acutely, Ms. Isaac has developed intense anxiety about leaving her apartment and entering the local supermarket. These symptoms suggest that Ms. Isaac may meet DSM-5 criteria for agoraphobia, which requires fears and avoidance of at least two different situations. Her agoraphobia symptoms have persisted only a few months, however, which is less than the 6-month DSM-5 requirement. Depending on whether the clinician thought the agoraphobia symptoms warranted clinical attention, Ms. Isaac could receive an additional diagnosis of "unspecified anxiety disorder (agoraphobia with inadequate duration of symptoms)."

In addition to making a DSM-5 diagnosis, it is also important to consider what might have precipitated Ms. Isaac's GAD. Although it is not possible to be certain why someone develops a mood or anxiety disorder, consideration of psychosocial stressors that are coincident with the onset of symptoms can help with formulation, goal setting, and treatment.

In this case, Ms. Isaac developed acute anxiety symptoms after her live-in boyfriend broke up with her and she moved into another apartment. Both of these events were acutely upsetting. The next part of answering "Why now?" involves thinking about how the stressors relate to long-standing issues in Ms. Isaac's life. She noted that she had "never [been] single for very long," and gave a history of difficulties with separation that began in childhood. Anxiety that is triggered by separation may suggest problems with attachment, and adult attachment styles are thought to be linked to the individual's earliest relationships. Those with secure attachments are able to form intimate relationships with others but are also able to soothe and regulate themselves when alone.

Individuals with insecure attachments, on the other hand, may cling to loved ones, be unable to self-regulate when alone, and have ambivalent feelings about those upon whom they are dependent. Thinking in this way, one can hypothesize that Ms. Isaac may have become symptomatic because of an insecure attachment style linked to her earliest relationship with her mother.

Clues that this may be the case include her mother's feeling that Ms. Isaac was "too clingy" during the divorce and Ms. Isaac's ambivalent feelings about her mother's efforts to be supportive. It would be helpful to understand more about Ms. Isaac's earliest relationships and the sorts of problematic attachment patterns that have developed during her romantic relationships. Such patterns would likely be recapitulated in the therapeutic relationship, where they could become a focus of treatment.

Suggested Readings

Blanco C, Rubio JM, Wall M, et al: The latent structure and comorbidity patterns of generalized anxiety disorder and major depressive disorder: a national study. Depress Anxiety June 14, 2013 [Epub ahead of print]

Stein DJ, Hollander E, Rothbaum BO (eds): Textbook of Anxiety Disorders, 2nd Edition. Washington, DC, American Psychiatric Publishing, 2009

Case 6: Anxiety and Cirrhosis

Andrea DiMartini, M.D.
Catherine Crone, M.D.

A psychiatric transplant liaison service was called to evaluate Robert Jennings, a 50-year-old married white man, for orthotopic liver transplant in the context of alcohol dependence, advanced cirrhosis, and no other prior psychiatric history. Several weeks earlier, he had been hospitalized with acute alcoholic hepatitis and diagnosed with end-stage liver disease. Prednisolone 40 mg/day was prescribed for treatment of his alcoholic hepatitis. Prior to that hospitalization, he had been unaware that his alcohol consumption was seriously damaging his health and was shocked to learn he would eventually require a liver transplant. Upon discharge, he began an addiction treatment program that was mandatory for him to be listed for possible transplantation.

Outpatient psychiatric consultation was requested by the transplant team after the patient's family expressed concern that he had recently become increasingly irritable and anxious and seemed to be having difficulty coping with the requirements for transplantation. Mr. Jennings's primary care physician had recently prescribed alprazolam 0.5 mg as needed for his anxiety. This was initially helpful, but after several days his family noticed he seemed more irritable, lethargic, and forgetful.

When interviewed, the patient said that he had been tired for months prior to the diagnosis and that the fatigue had hampered his ability to work making deliveries for a shipping firm. Although the diagnosis had been a shock, he said he had felt "great" when he first left the hospital, with enhanced energy and sense of well-being. About 1 week after discharge, however, he began to feel anxious and restless. He could not concentrate or sleep well and worried constantly about his health, finances, and family. He became less engaged with his family and stopped watching movies, normally enjoyable activities.

He denied having nightmares, flashbacks, avoidant behaviors, or racing thoughts. He also denied low mood, tearfulness, appetite changes, anhedonia, helplessness, hopelessness, or suicidality. He admitted feeling occasionally guilty over his alcohol use and its impact on him and his family. He denied using any alcohol since his hospitalization. He admitted to anger over having to undergo addiction counseling and had argued with the transplant team about this requirement. In the past, he had considered himself able to handle most of life's challenges without being overwhelmed. His family confirmed his description of himself and viewed his recent behavior as uncharacteristic.

On mental status examination, Mr. Jennings was a thin, tired-appearing, slightly jaundiced man. His gait was normal, but he was fidgety while seated. He maintained eye contact and responded appropriately, although he repeatedly made comments like, "Something isn't right" and "It's not all in my head." His affect was anxious and irritable, and his speech was terse. He appeared distracted but denied confusion and disorientation. He had no delusions or hallucinations. His thoughts were logical and coherent, without disorganization, and there was no latency to his responses. He scored 26 out of 30 on the Mini-Mental State Examination (MMSE), missing points for recall and serial 7s. He scored in the normal range for Trail Making Tests A and B but asked to have the instructions repeated for Trails B.

Diagnoses

- Alcohol use disorder
- Medication-induced anxiety disorder (steroids)

Discussion

Mr. Jennings has been fatigued for several months. Diagnosis and treatment of his hepatic cirrhosis were followed by a weeklong burst of euphoria, followed by anxiety, depression, irritability, cognitive disturbances, and insomnia. The evaluating team would look broadly for causes of Mr. Jennings's psychiatric complaints, but the initial search would focus on medical causes. Liver disease rarely induces anxiety directly, but steroid therapy frequently induces an initial sense of well-being, followed within 1–2 weeks by more negative or unpleasant symptoms of mood or anxiety disturbance.

Other diagnoses should also be considered. Fatigue, difficulty concentrating, and a reduction in pleasurable activities point to the possibility of major depressive disorder, for example, although some of these symptoms could be attributable to progressive physical limitations from his advanced liver disease. Utilizing a broad or "inclusive" approach to the diagnosis of depression in medically ill patients might suggest that these symptoms be counted under the DSM-5 diagnostic criteria for major depressive disorder despite their potential physical origin. However, further review of the patient's presentation indicated no problems with persistent low mood, tearfulness, or other associated depressive symptoms (e.g., anhedonia, persistent insomnia, appetite changes, inappropriate thoughts of guilt, or recurrent thoughts of death or suicide). Major depression would seem unlikely.

Anxiety disorders such as generalized anxiety disorder and panic disorder should also be considered. The patient's symptoms seem directly related to the steroids, however, and the symptoms lack the duration to qualify for one of the other anxiety disorders.

Illness, treatments, and potentially life-threatening circumstances can lead to acute stress disorder, adjustment disorder, and posttraumatic stress disorder. This particular patient does not, however, appear to fulfill criteria for a trauma disorder. Furthermore, it is of note that he initially felt well despite his diagnosis and only later developed changes in his mood and behavior. This pattern would not rule out a trauma diagnosis but reduces the likelihood.

An additionally important diagnostic area to consider is Mr. Jennings's dependence on alcohol. Early in abstinence, patients often experience symptoms of anxiety, irritability, and depression. These symptoms contribute to the high rates of relapse following alcohol rehabilitation. Even in the context of life-threatening illness and the need for transplantation, a significant number of individuals will relapse. This particular patient has also started taking benzodiazepines, which can produce cravings and precipitate relapse. This patient is denying alcohol use, but he is on a transplant list, and a relapse could lead to a delisting. To monitor unrevealed alcohol use, it would be warranted to monitor him by ongoing interviews and random toxicology screenings.

Mr. Jennings's current presentation could also be related to a neurocognitive disorder. Patients with advanced liver disease frequently have problems with minimal hepatic encephalopathy, a phenomenon that is characterized by subtle but important changes in both physical and mental functioning. Compared with hepatic encephalopathy (DSM-5 delirium due to another medical condition), minimal hepatic encephalopathy does not present with disturbance of consciousness or with overt behavioral or cognitive functioning changes. Rather, patients may present with mild personality or behavioral changes such as irritability, excessive fatigue, or sleepiness, along with subtle subcortical cognitive impairment or slowing. Impairments in psychomotor speed, visual attention, and perception are typically not evident with basic screening such as the MMSE but require specific psychometric testing that would elicit these deficits (e.g., Trail Making Tests A and B, Digit Span, finger-tapping speed).

Identifying minimal hepatic encephalopathy is important because patients with this diagnosis typically do not improve with the use of antidepressants or anxiolytics but instead require treatment with ammonia-reducing agents. The combination of minimal hepatic encephalopathy and slower hepatic metabolism makes patients more sensitive to adverse drug side effects (e.g., cognitive slowing from benzodiazepines, sedatives, pain medications, or anticholinergic medications). In Mr. Jennings's case, the worsening of symptoms may have resulted from the use of a benzodiazepine. These patients need to avoid medications that may worsen cognitive functioning, and they should also be monitored for development of overt hepatic encephalopathy. Because cognitive difficulties that accompany minimal hepatic encephalopathy are known to impair daily functioning and skills such as driving, this patient may need to be counseled on whether he can or should continue to drive (which would have significant implications for his work as a deliveryman). After discontinuing the alprazolam and receiving treatment for high ammonia levels (if present), he could be retested to establish his cognitive baseline.

Suggested Readings

DiMartini A, Crone C, Fireman M, et al: Psychiatric aspects of organ transplantation in critical care. Crit Care Clin 24(4):949–981, 2008

DiMartini A, Dew MA, Crone C: Organ transplantation, in Kaplan & Sadock's Comprehensive Textbook of Psychiatry, 9th Edition, Vol 2. Edited by Sadock B, Sadock VA, Ruiz P. Philadelphia, PA, Lippincott Williams & Wilkins, 2009, pp 2441–2456

Dubovsky AN, Arvikar S, Stern TA, et al: The neuropsychiatric complications of glucocorticoid use: steroid psychosis revisited. Psychosomatics 53(2):103–115, 2012

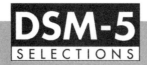

Anxiety Disorders

DSM-5® Self-Exam Questions

1. Which of the following disorders is included in the "Anxiety Disorders" chapter of DSM-5?

   A. Obsessive-compulsive disorder.
   B. Posttraumatic stress disorder.
   C. Acute stress disorder.
   D. Panic disorder with agoraphobia.
   E. Separation anxiety disorder.

2. A 9-year-old boy cannot go to sleep without having a parent in his room. While falling asleep, he frequently awakens to check that a parent is still there. One parent usually stays until the boy falls asleep. If he wakes up alone during the night, he starts to panic and gets up to find his parents. He also reports frequent nightmares in which he or his parents are harmed. He occasionally calls out that he saw a strange figure peering into his dark room. The parents usually wake in the morning to find the boy asleep on the floor of their room. They once tried to leave him with a relative so they could go on a vacation; however, he became so distressed in anticipation of this that they canceled their plans. What is the most likely diagnosis?

   A. Specific phobia.
   B. Nightmare disorder.
   C. Delusional disorder.
   D. Separation anxiety disorder.
   E. Agoraphobia.

3. Which of the following is considered a culture-specific symptom of panic attacks?

   A. Derealization.
   B. Headaches.
   C. Fear of going crazy.
   D. Shortness of breath.
   E. Heat sensations.

4. Which of the following statements best describes how panic attacks differ from panic disorder?

    A. Panic attacks require fewer symptoms for a definitive diagnosis.
    B. Panic attacks are discrete, occur suddenly, and are usually less severe.
    C. Panic attacks are invariably unexpected.
    D. Panic attacks represent a syndrome that can occur with a variety of other disorders.
    E. Panic attacks cannot be secondary to a medical condition.

5. The determination of whether a panic attack is expected or unexpected is ultimately best made by which of the following?

    A. Careful clinical judgment.
    B. Whether the patient associates it with external stress.
    C. The presence or absence of nocturnal panic attacks.
    D. Ruling out possible culture-specific syndromes.
    E. 24-Hour electroencephalographic monitoring.

6. A 50-year-old man reports episodes in which he suddenly and unexpectedly awakens from sleep feeling a surge of intense fear that peaks within minutes. During this time, he feels short of breath and has heart palpitations, sweating, and nausea. His medical history is significant only for hypertension, which is well controlled with hydrochlorothiazide. As a result of these symptoms, he has begun to have anticipatory anxiety associated with going to sleep. What is the most likely explanation for his symptoms?

    A. Anxiety disorder due to another medical condition (hypertension).
    B. Substance/medication-induced anxiety disorder.
    C. Panic disorder.
    D. Sleep terrors.
    E. Panic attacks.

7. A 32-year-old woman reports sudden, unexpected episodes of intense anxiety, accompanied by headaches, a rapid pulse, nausea, and shortness of breath. During the episodes she fears that she is dying, and she has presented several times to emergency departments. Each time she has been told that she is medically healthy; she is usually reassured for a time, but on the occurrence of a new episode she again becomes concerned that she has some severe medical problem. She was given lorazepam once but disliked the sedating effect and has not taken it again. She abstains from all medications and alcohol in an attempt to minimize potential causes for her attacks. What is the most likely explanation for her symptoms?

    A. Panic disorder.
    B. Somatic symptom disorder.
    C. Anxiety due to another medical condition.

    D. Illness anxiety disorder.

    E. Specific phobia.

8. A 65-year-old woman reports being housebound despite feeling physically healthy. Several years ago, she fell while shopping; although she sustained no injuries, the situation was so upsetting that she became extremely nervous when she had to leave her house unaccompanied. Because she has no children and few friends whom she can ask to accompany her, she is very distressed that she has few opportunities to venture outside her home. What is the most likely diagnosis?

    A. Specific phobia, situational type.

    B. Social anxiety disorder (social phobia).

    C. Posttraumatic stress disorder.

    D. Agoraphobia.

    E. Adjustment disorder.

9. A 32-year-old man has regularly experienced panic attacks when out of his home alone and when on the bus. He now avoids leaving home for fear of experiencing these attacks. What is the most appropriate diagnosis?

    A. Panic disorder with agoraphobia.

    B. Agoraphobia with panic attacks.

    C. Specific phobia, situational type.

    D. Two separate disorders: panic disorder and agoraphobia.

    E. Delusional disorder.

10. A 35-year-old man is in danger of losing his job because it requires frequent long-range traveling and for the past year he has avoided flying. Two years earlier he was on a particularly turbulent flight, and although he was not in any real danger, he was convinced that the pilot minimized the risk and that the plane almost crashed. He flew again 1 month later and, despite having a smooth flight, the anticipation of turbulence was so distressing that he experienced a panic attack during the flight; he has not flown since. What is the most appropriate diagnosis?

    A. Agoraphobia.

    B. Acute stress disorder.

    C. Specific phobia, situational type.

    D. Social anxiety disorder (social phobia).

    E. Panic disorder.

11. Which of the following types of specific phobia is most likely to be associated with vasovagal fainting?

    A. Animal type.

    B. Natural environment type.

    C. Blood-injection-injury type.
    D. Situational type.
    E. Other (e.g., in children, loud sounds or costumed characters).

12. Which of the following most accurately describes people with specific phobias?

    A. The average individual with a phobia has fears of only one object or situation.
    B. The fear is usually quite mild in intensity.
    C. Fewer than 10% of people fear more than one object or situation.
    D. The fear occurs almost every time the person encounters the object or situation.
    E. The fear is exactly the same in intensity each time the object or situation is encountered.

13. Although onset of a specific phobia can occur at any age, specific phobia most typically develops during which age period?

    A. Childhood.
    B. Late adolescence to early adulthood.
    C. Middle age.
    D. Old age.
    E. Any age.

14. In social anxiety disorder (social phobia), the object of an individual's fear is the potential for which of the following?

    A. Social or occupational impairment.
    B. Harm to self or others.
    C. Embarrassment.
    D. Separation from objects of attachment.
    E. Incapacitating symptoms.

15. When called on at school, a 7-year-old boy will only nod or write in response. The family of the child is surprised to hear this from the teacher, because the boy speaks normally when at home with his parents. The child has achieved appropriate developmental milestones, and a medical evaluation indicates that he is healthy. The boy is unable to give any explanation for his behavior, but the parents are concerned that it will affect his school performance. What diagnosis best fits this child's symptoms?

    A. Separation anxiety disorder.
    B. Autism spectrum disorder.
    C. Agoraphobia.
    D. Selective mutism.
    E. Communication disorder.

16. Social anxiety disorder (social phobia) differs from normative shyness in that the disorder leads to which of the following?

    A. Social or occupational dysfunction.
    B. Marked social reticence.
    C. Avoidance of social situations.
    D. Derealization or depersonalization.
    E. Pervasive social deficits with poor insight.

17. In addition to feeling restless or "keyed up," individuals with generalized anxiety disorder are most likely to experience which of the following symptoms?

    A. Panic attacks.
    B. Obsessions.
    C. Muscle tension.
    D. Multiple somatic complaints.
    E. Social anxiety.

18. Which of the following characteristics of generalized anxiety disorder is especially common in children who have the disorder?

    A. Complaining of physical aches and pains.
    B. Excessively preparing for activities.
    C. Avoiding activities that may provoke anxiety.
    D. Seeking frequent reassurance from others.
    E. Delaying or procrastinating before activities.

19. What is the primary difference in the clinical expression of generalized anxiety disorder across age groups?

    A. Content of worry.
    B. Degree of worry.
    C. Patterns of comorbidity.
    D. Predominance of cognitive versus somatic symptoms.
    E. Severity of impairment.

20. In what aspect of generalized anxiety disorder do men and women most commonly differ?

    A. Course.
    B. Symptom profile.
    C. Degree of impairment.
    D. Patterns of comorbidity.
    E. Age at onset.

21. Which of the following is more suggestive of anxiety that is not pathological than of anxiety that qualifies for a diagnosis of generalized anxiety disorder?

    A. Anxiety and worry that interferes significantly with functioning.
    B. Anxiety and worry that lasts for months to years.
    C. Anxiety and worry in response to a clear precipitant.
    D. Anxiety and worry focused on a wide range of life circumstances.
    E. Anxiety and worry accompanied by physical symptoms.

22. A 26-year-old man is brought to the emergency department suffering from a sudden, severe surge of panic. He has no history of panic disorder, but he reports taking several doses of an over-the-counter cold medication earlier that day. Which of the following clinical features, if present in this case, would help to confirm a diagnosis of substance/medication-induced anxiety disorder?

    A. Symptoms that are mild and do not impair functioning.
    B. Symptoms that persist for a long time after substance/medication use.
    C. Symptoms that are in excess of what would be expected for the substance/medication.
    D. Presence of a delirium or gross confusion.
    E. Lack of any history of anxiety disorder or panic symptoms.

23. In which of the following circumstances would a diagnosis of substance/medication-induced anxiety disorder be appropriate for an individual who stopped taking benzodiazepines the previous day?

    A. Significant anxiety symptoms are present.
    B. Anxiety is present that is clearly related to the withdrawal state.
    C. Anxiety is present that is sufficiently severe to warrant independent clinical attention.
    D. Anxiety is present only during bouts of delirium.
    E. Never: the diagnosis of substance withdrawal would supersede the anxiety disorder diagnosis.

24. A 60-year-old man has just been diagnosed with congestive heart failure. He is intensely anxious and reports feeling as if he cannot breathe, which causes him to panic. Which of the following features, if present in this case, would tend to support a diagnosis of anxiety disorder due to another medical condition rather than adjustment disorder with anxiety?

    A. The patient says that he is relieved to know his diagnosis.
    B. The patient has no anxiety-associated physical symptoms.
    C. The patient is focused on the reasons he has a cardiac disorder.
    D. The patient is delirious.
    E. The patient is extremely concerned that he will not be able to return to work.

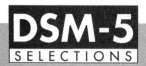

Anxiety Disorders
DSM-5® Self-Exam Answer Guide

1. Which of the following disorders is included in the "Anxiety Disorders" chapter of DSM-5?

    A. Obsessive-compulsive disorder.
    B. Posttraumatic stress disorder.
    C. Acute stress disorder.
    D. Panic disorder with agoraphobia.
    E. Separation anxiety disorder.

    Correct Answer: E. Separation anxiety disorder.

    Explanation: The DSM-5 "Anxiety Disorders" chapter contains a number of additions and deletions when compared with the prior edition. A number of anxiety disorders classified by DSM-IV as disorders usually first diagnosed in infancy, childhood, or adolescence are now included among the DSM-5 anxiety disorders, including separation anxiety disorder and selective mutism. Several DSM-IV disorders from the "Anxiety Disorders" chapter, including obsessive-compulsive disorder, posttraumatic stress disorder, and acute stress disorder, were removed from that section in DSM-5. This reorganization was the result of a scientific review that concluded that these were distinct disorders that were not sufficiently described by the presence of anxiety symptoms. Agoraphobia has been separated from panic disorder as a distinct disorder in DSM-5, which includes a panic attack specifier when they co-occur.

    1—Chapter intro (pp. 189–190)

2. A 9-year-old boy cannot go to sleep without having a parent in his room. While falling asleep, he frequently awakens to check that a parent is still there. One parent usually stays until the boy falls asleep. If he wakes up alone during the night, he starts to panic and gets up to find his parents. He also reports frequent nightmares in which he or his parents are harmed. He occasionally calls out that he saw a strange figure peering into his dark room. The parents usually wake in the morning to find the boy asleep on the floor of their room. They once tried to leave him with a relative so they could go on a vacation; however, he became so distressed in anticipation of this that they canceled their plans. What is the most likely diagnosis?

A. Specific phobia.
B. Nightmare disorder.
C. Delusional disorder.
D. Separation anxiety disorder.
E. Agoraphobia.

Correct Answer: D. Separation anxiety disorder.

Explanation: The essential feature of separation anxiety disorder is excessive anxiety about being separated from home or attachment figures, beyond what would be expected for the person's developmental stage. By definition, it firsts presents before age 18; however, it may continue into adulthood. Typical presentations include reluctance to leave home or even stay in a room without a parent. In the latter case, children frequently have difficulty at bedtime and may insist that a parent stay with them. They frequently express fear of harm or untoward events that may prevent them from being with a loved one, and they may have nightmares regarding these fears as well as unusual perceptual experiences, particularly at night or in the dark. Although the other disorders listed should be ruled out, the child's focus on a fear of being left alone makes separation anxiety disorder the most likely diagnosis.

2—Separation Anxiety Disorder / Diagnostic Features (pp. 191–192)

3. Which of the following is considered a culture-specific symptom of panic attacks?

A. Derealization.
B. Headaches.
C. Fear of going crazy.
D. Shortness of breath.
E. Heat sensations.

Correct Answer: B. Headaches.

Explanation: All of the symptoms listed may occur as part of a panic attack. Culture-specific symptoms (e.g., tinnitus, neck soreness, headache, and uncontrollable screaming or crying) may be seen; however, such symptoms should not count as one of the four required symptoms. Frequency of each of the 13 symptoms varies cross-culturally (e.g., higher rates of paresthesias in African Americans and of dizziness in several Asian groups). Cultural syndromes also influence the cross-cultural presentation of panic attacks, resulting in different symptom profiles across different cultural groups. Examples include *khyâl* (wind) attacks, a Cambodian cultural syndrome involving dizziness, tinnitus, and neck soreness; and *trúng gió* (wind-related) attacks, a Vietnamese cultural syndrome associated with headaches.

3—Panic Attack Specifier / Culture-Related Diagnostic Issues (p. 216)

4. Which of the following statements best describes how panic attacks differ from panic disorder?

   A. Panic attacks require fewer symptoms for a definitive diagnosis.
   B. Panic attacks are discrete, occur suddenly, and are usually less severe.
   C. Panic attacks are invariably unexpected.
   D. Panic attacks represent a syndrome that can occur with a variety of other disorders.
   E. Panic attacks cannot be secondary to a medical condition.

   Correct Answer: D. Panic attacks represent a syndrome that can occur with a variety of other disorders.

   Explanation: Panic attacks are abrupt surges of intense fear or intense discomfort that reach a peak within minutes, accompanied by physical and/or cognitive symptoms. Panic attacks may be either *expected* (e.g., in response to a typically feared object or situation) or *unexpected* (meaning that the panic attack occurs for no apparent reason). Although DSM-5 defines symptoms for the purpose of identifying a panic attack, panic attack is not a mental disorder and cannot be coded. Panic attacks can occur in the context of any anxiety disorder as well as other mental disorders (e.g., depressive disorders, posttraumatic stress disorder, substance use disorders) and some medical conditions (e.g., cardiac, respiratory, vestibular, gastrointestinal). When the presence of a panic attack is identified, it should be noted as a specifier (e.g., "posttraumatic stress disorder with panic attacks"). For panic disorder, the presence of panic attack is contained within the criteria for the disorder, and panic attack is not used as a specifier.

   4—Chapter intro (pp. 190–191); Panic Attack Specifier /specifier description (p. 214); Features (pp. 214–215)

5. The determination of whether a panic attack is expected or unexpected is ultimately best made by which of the following?

   A. Careful clinical judgment.
   B. Whether the patient associates it with external stress.
   C. The presence or absence of nocturnal panic attacks.
   D. Ruling out possible culture-specific syndromes.
   E. 24-Hour electroencephalographic monitoring.

   Correct Answer: A. Careful clinical judgment.

   Explanation: It can be difficult to determine whether panic attacks are expected (i.e., triggered by some external stress or situation). Patients (particularly older individuals) may retrospectively attribute panic attacks to certain stressful situations even if they were unexpected in the moment. Laboratory testing may rule out other potential medical causes. Agents with disparate mechanisms of action, such as sodium lactate, caffeine, isoproterenol, yohimbine, carbon dioxide, or cholecystokinin, provoke panic attacks in individuals with panic disorder to a much greater extent than in healthy control subjects (and in some cases, than in individuals with other anxiety, depressive, or bipolar disorders without panic attacks). In a proportion of individuals with panic disorder, panic attacks are related to hypersensitive medullary carbon dioxide detectors, resulting in hypocapnia and other respiratory irregularities; however, none of these laboratory findings are considered diagnostic of panic disorder. There is no definitive test; ultimately the determination is based on a clinical judgment that takes into account the sequence of events leading to the attack, the patient's own sense of whether triggers are present, and potential cultural factors that may influence a determination of cause.

5—Panic Attack Specifier / Features (pp. 214–215)

6. A 50-year-old man reports episodes in which he suddenly and unexpectedly awakens from sleep feeling a surge of intense fear that peaks within minutes. During this time, he feels short of breath and has heart palpitations, sweating, and nausea. His medical history is significant only for hypertension, which is well controlled with hydrochlorothiazide. As a result of these symptoms, he has begun to have anticipatory anxiety associated with going to sleep. What is the most likely explanation for his symptoms?

   A. Anxiety disorder due to another medical condition (hypertension).
   B. Substance/medication-induced anxiety disorder.
   C. Panic disorder.
   D. Sleep terrors.
   E. Panic attacks.

Correct Answer: C. Panic disorder.

Explanation: Panic disorder involves recurrent, unexpected panic attacks. Panic attacks are a syndrome, not a disorder, and can occur with a variety of disorders. Other medical conditions, substance-related disorders, and other psychiatric disorders must be ruled out; in this vignette, the patient's well-controlled hypertension and use of a diuretic are unlikely to be the cause of his attacks. Nocturnal panic attacks associated with sleep are an example of an unexpected panic attack. Although sleep-related disorders should be ruled out, this classic presentation makes panic disorder the most likely explanation.

6—Panic Disorder / diagnostic criteria; Diagnostic Features (p. 209)

7. A 32-year-old woman reports sudden, unexpected episodes of intense anxiety, accompanied by headaches, a rapid pulse, nausea, and shortness of breath. During the episodes she fears that she is dying, and she has presented several

times to emergency departments. Each time she has been told that she is medically healthy; she is usually reassured for a time, but on the occurrence of a new episode she again becomes concerned that she has some severe medical problem. She was given lorazepam once but disliked the sedating effect and has not taken it again. She abstains from all medications and alcohol in an attempt to minimize potential causes for her attacks. What is the most likely explanation for her symptoms?

A. Panic disorder.
B. Somatic symptom disorder.
C. Anxiety due to another medical condition.
D. Illness anxiety disorder.
E. Specific phobia.

Correct Answer: A. Panic disorder.

Explanation: The presence of sudden, unexpected panic attacks in the absence of a medical disorder is the main feature of panic disorder. In addition to worries about the attacks, many individuals report broader concerns about health and mental health outcomes. In a search for an explanation for their symptoms, they may worry about having a major disease. This differs from illness anxiety disorder in that the concern with panic attacks stems from what might be seen as a reasonable concern over their dramatic and unexplained symptoms; patients with panic attacks do not show the preoccupation with having a feared disease that is typical of illness anxiety disorder (or hypochondriasis in DSM-IV). Specific phobia refers to anxiety centered on a specific trigger.

7—Panic Disorder / Differential Diagnosis (pp. 212–213)

8. A 65-year-old woman reports being housebound despite feeling physically healthy. Several years ago, she fell while shopping; although she sustained no injuries, the situation was so upsetting that she became extremely nervous when she had to leave her house unaccompanied. Because she has no children and few friends whom she can ask to accompany her, she is very distressed that she has few opportunities to venture outside her home. What is the most likely diagnosis?

A. Specific phobia, situational type.
B. Social anxiety disorder (social phobia).
C. Posttraumatic stress disorder.
D. Agoraphobia.
E. Adjustment disorder.

Correct Answer: D. Agoraphobia.

Explanation: The essential feature of agoraphobia is marked fear or anxiety triggered by real or anticipated exposure to a variety of situations (e.g., using public transportation, going to open or public spaces) from which escape or help might not be available. DSM-IV treated agoraphobia as a feature of panic disorder, and individuals do frequently report a fear of having a panic attack in the dreaded situations; however, there are other incapacitating situations that could cause similar fear, including a fear of falling or of incontinence. This disorder can be very similar to other phobias such as social anxiety disorder (social phobia) and specific phobia, situational type; however, the focus of the fear is not the situation itself, but rather the fear that an incapacitating event may occur during the situation. Agoraphobia does not have the cluster of symptoms associated with posttraumatic stress disorder and is not merely indicative of poor adjustment to a uniquely stressful situation.

8—Agoraphobia / diagnostic criteria; Diagnostic Features (pp. 217–219)

9. A 32-year-old man has regularly experienced panic attacks when out of his home alone and when on the bus. He now avoids leaving home for fear of experiencing these attacks. What is the most appropriate diagnosis?

    A. Panic disorder with agoraphobia.
    B. Agoraphobia with panic attacks.
    C. Specific phobia, situational type.
    D. Two separate disorders: panic disorder and agoraphobia.
    E. Delusional disorder.

Correct Answer: D. Two separate disorders: panic disorder and agoraphobia.

Explanation: This man has panic disorder, not just panic attacks, and he also has agoraphobia. Whereas DSM-IV considered the co-occurrence of panic and agoraphobia as a subtype of panic attacks, agoraphobia with or without panic is now a separate diagnosis; the presence of panic attacks can be indicated by a specifier. In specific phobia, the fear would be of the situation itself rather than the possibility of having a panic attack.

9—Agoraphobia / diagnostic criteria / Diagnostic Features (pp. 217–219)

10. A 35-year-old man is in danger of losing his job because it requires frequent long-range traveling and for the past year he has avoided flying. Two years earlier he was on a particularly turbulent flight, and although he was not in any real danger, he was convinced that the pilot minimized the risk and that the plane almost crashed. He flew again 1 month later and, despite having a smooth flight, the anticipation of turbulence was so distressing that he experienced a panic attack during the flight; he has not flown since. What is the most appropriate diagnosis?

    A. Agoraphobia.
    B. Acute stress disorder.
    C. Specific phobia, situational type.

D. Social anxiety disorder (social phobia).

E. Panic disorder.

Correct Answer: C. Specific phobia, situational type.

Explanation: Specific phobia is characterized by the marked fear or anxiety of a specific object or situation, which is perceived as being dangerous. This differs from agoraphobia, in which the focus of the anxiety is on the possibility of having panic or other incapacitating symptoms, or social anxiety disorder in which the focus is on being scrutinized by others. Trauma-related disorders should be considered in the differential diagnosis; however, the lack of any real danger makes this unlikely, and the time course is not compatible with the criteria for acute stress disorder. Although the man did experience a panic attack, patients with many disorders, including specific phobia, can experience such attacks. Panic disorder should be diagnosed only when the attacks are unexpected and not otherwise explained by other disorders.

10—Specific Phobia / diagnostic criteria; Diagnostic Features (pp. 197–199)

11. Which of the following types of specific phobia is most likely to be associated with vasovagal fainting?

    A. Animal type.

    B. Natural environment type.

    C. Blood-injection-injury type.

    D. Situational type.

    E. Other (e.g., in children, loud sounds or costumed characters).

Correct Answer: C. Blood-injection-injury type.

Explanation: Whereas most phobias show a profile of sympathetic nervous system arousal, individuals with blood-injection-injury phobias often demonstrate vasovagal fainting or near-fainting marked by brief increases in heart rate and blood pressure, followed by subsequent rapid decreases of both.

11—Specific Phobia / Associated Features Supporting Diagnosis (p. 199)

12. Which of the following most accurately describes people with specific phobias?

    A. The average individual with a phobia has fears of only one object or situation.

    B. The fear is usually quite mild in intensity.

    C. Fewer than 10% of people fear more than one object or situation.

    D. The fear occurs almost every time the person encounters the object or situation.

    E. The fear is exactly the same in intensity each time the object or situation is encountered.

Correct Answer: D. The fear occurs almost every time the person encounters the object or situation.

Explanation: A key feature of specific phobia is that the fear or anxiety is circumscribed to the presence of a particular situation or object (Criterion A), which may be termed the *phobic stimulus*. Categories of feared situations or objects (i.e., *phobic stimuli*) are provided as specifiers in the diagnostic criteria. Many individuals fear objects or situations from more than one category. For the diagnosis of specific phobia, the response must differ from normal, transient fears that commonly occur in the population. To meet the criteria for a diagnosis, the fear or anxiety must be intense or severe (i.e., "marked"; Criterion A). The amount of fear experienced may vary with proximity to the feared object or situation and may occur in anticipation of or in the actual presence of the object or situation. Also, the fear or anxiety may take the form of a full or limited-symptom panic attack (i.e., expected panic attack). Another characteristic of specific phobias is that fear or anxiety is evoked nearly every time the individual comes into contact with the phobic stimulus (Criterion B). Thus, an individual who becomes anxious only occasionally upon being confronted with the situation or object (e.g., becomes anxious when flying only on one out of every five airplane flights) would not be diagnosed with specific phobia. However, the degree of fear or anxiety expressed may vary (from anticipatory anxiety to a full panic attack) across different occasions of encountering the phobic object or situation because of various contextual factors, such as the presence of others, duration of exposure, and other threatening elements such as turbulence on a flight for individuals who fear flying.

12—Specific Phobia / Specifiers; Diagnostic Features (pp. 198–199)

13. Although onset of a specific phobia can occur at any age, specific phobia most typically develops during which age period?

    A. Childhood.
    B. Late adolescence to early adulthood.
    C. Middle age.
    D. Old age.
    E. Any age.

Correct Answer: A. Childhood.

Explanation: Specific phobia usually develops in early childhood, with the majority of cases developing prior to age 10 years. The median age at onset is between 7 and 11 years, with the mean at about 10 years. *Situational* specific phobias tend to have a later age at onset than do *natural environment, animal,* or *blood-injection-injury* specific phobias. Specific phobias that develop in childhood and adolescence are likely to wax and wane during that period. However, phobias that persist into adulthood are unlikely to remit for the majority of individuals.

When specific phobia is being diagnosed in children, two issues should be considered. First, young children may express their fear and anxiety by crying, tantrums, freezing, or clinging. Second, young children typically are not able to understand the concept of avoidance. Therefore, the clinician should assemble additional information from parents, teachers, or others who know the child well.

13—Specific Phobia / Development and Course (pp. 199–200)

14. In social anxiety disorder (social phobia), the object of an individual's fear is the potential for which of the following?

    A. Social or occupational impairment.
    B. Harm to self or others.
    C. Embarrassment.
    D. Separation from objects of attachment.
    E. Incapacitating symptoms.

Correct Answer: C. Embarrassment.

Explanation: The anxiety disorders differ in the object or cause of an individual's fear. In the case of social anxiety disorder, an individual experiences fear or anxiety in situations in which he or she is exposed to scrutiny; the fear is that this may result in humiliation, embarrassment, or offense to others. In contrast, individuals with specific phobia fear harmful objects, animals, or situations; individuals with separation anxiety fear being away from home or loved ones; and individuals with agoraphobia avoid situations in which the individual might have panic-like or other incapacitating symptoms. In all cases, the disorders cause significant social or occupational impairment; however, this impairment is the result rather than the object of the fear.

14—Social Anxiety Disorder (Social Phobia) / diagnostic criteria (pp. 202–203)

15. When called on at school, a 7-year-old boy will only nod or write in response. The family of the child is surprised to hear this from the teacher, because the boy speaks normally when at home with his parents. The child has achieved appropriate developmental milestones, and a medical evaluation indicates that he is healthy. The boy is unable to give any explanation for his behavior, but the parents are concerned that it will affect his school performance. What diagnosis best fits this child's symptoms?

    A. Separation anxiety disorder.
    B. Autism spectrum disorder.
    C. Agoraphobia.
    D. Selective mutism.
    E. Communication disorder.

Correct Answer: D. Selective mutism.

Explanation: When encountering other individuals in social interactions, children with selective mutism do not initiate speech or reciprocally respond when spoken to. Lack of speech occurs in social interactions with children or adults. Children with selective mutism will speak in their home in the presence of immediate family members but often not even in front of close friends or second-degree relatives, such as grandparents or cousins. The disturbance is often marked by high social anxiety. Children with selective mutism often refuse to speak at school, leading to academic or educational impairment, as teachers often find it difficult to assess skills such as reading. The lack of speech may interfere with social communication, although children with this disorder sometimes use nonspoken or nonverbal means (e.g., grunting, pointing, writing) to communicate and may be willing or eager to perform or engage in social encounters when speech is not required (e.g., nonverbal parts in school plays).

15—Selective Mutism / Diagnostic Features (p. 195)

16. Social anxiety disorder (social phobia) differs from normative shyness in that the disorder leads to which of the following?

    A. Social or occupational dysfunction.
    B. Marked social reticence.
    C. Avoidance of social situations.
    D. Derealization or depersonalization.
    E. Pervasive social deficits with poor insight.

Correct Answer: A. Social or occupational dysfunction.

Explanation: Shyness (i.e., social reticence) is a common personality trait and is not by itself pathological. In some societies, shyness is even evaluated positively. However, when there is a significant adverse impact on social, occupational, and other important areas of functioning, a diagnosis of social anxiety disorder should be considered, and when full diagnostic criteria for social anxiety disorder are met, the disorder should be diagnosed. Only a minority (12%) of self-identified shy individuals in the United States have symptoms that meet diagnostic criteria for social anxiety disorder.

16—Social Anxiety Disorder (Social Phobia) / Differential Diagnosis (pp. 206–207)

17. In addition to feeling restless or "keyed up," individuals with generalized anxiety disorder are most likely to experience which of the following symptoms?

    A. Panic attacks.
    B. Obsessions.
    C. Muscle tension.
    D. Multiple somatic complaints.
    E. Social anxiety.

Correct Answer: C. Muscle tension.

Explanation: Generalized anxiety disorder is defined as excessive anxiety and worry that occurs more days than not, lasts for at least 6 months, and is associated with restlessness or feeling keyed up or on edge and muscle tension. The anxiety cannot be due to other anxiety disorders; the symptoms listed in the other options suggest other disorders that would be part of the differential diagnosis (i.e., panic disorder [option A], obsessive-compulsive disorder [option B], somatic symptom disorder [option D], and social anxiety disorder [social phobia] [option E]).

17—Generalized Anxiety Disorder / diagnostic criteria (p. 222)

18. Which of the following characteristics of generalized anxiety disorder is especially common in children who have the disorder?

   A. Complaining of physical aches and pains.
   B. Excessively preparing for activities.
   C. Avoiding activities that may provoke anxiety.
   D. Seeking frequent reassurance from others.
   E. Delaying or procrastinating before activities.

Correct Answer: D. Seeking frequent reassurance from others.

Explanation: All of the behaviors listed are typical of generalized anxiety disorder; however, seeking reassurance from others (i.e., friends, family, practitioners) is especially common in children.

18—Generalized Anxiety Disorder / Development and Course (pp. 223–224)

19. What is the primary difference in the clinical expression of generalized anxiety disorder across age groups?

   A. Content of worry.
   B. Degree of worry.
   C. Patterns of comorbidity.
   D. Predominance of cognitive versus somatic symptoms.
   E. Severity of impairment.

Correct Answer: A. Content of worry.

Explanation: The clinical expression of generalized anxiety disorder is relatively consistent across the life span and the primary difference across age groups is the content of an individual's worry. Children and adolescents tend to worry about school or sports performance, whereas adults are more likely to be concerned about their personal health or the well-being of their family.

19—Generalized Anxiety Disorder / Development and Course (pp. 223–224)

20. In what aspect of generalized anxiety disorder do men and women most commonly differ?

    A. Course.
    B. Symptom profile.
    C. Degree of impairment.
    D. Patterns of comorbidity.
    E. Age at onset.

Correct Answer: D. Patterns of comorbidity.

Explanation: Women and men with generalized anxiety disorder tend to have similar symptoms and presentation; however, they have different patterns of comorbidity consistent with gender differences in the prevalence of mental disorders.

20—Generalized Anxiety Disorder / Gender-Related Diagnostic Issues (pp. 224–225)

21. Which of the following is more suggestive of anxiety that is not pathological than of anxiety that qualifies for a diagnosis of generalized anxiety disorder?

    A. Anxiety and worry that interferes significantly with functioning.
    B. Anxiety and worry that lasts for months to years.
    C. Anxiety and worry in response to a clear precipitant.
    D. Anxiety and worry focused on a wide range of life circumstances.
    E. Anxiety and worry accompanied by physical symptoms.

Correct Answer: C. Anxiety and worry in response to a clear precipitant.

Explanation: Several features distinguish generalized anxiety disorder from anxiety that is not pathological. First, the worries associated with generalized anxiety disorder are more pervasive, pronounced, and distressing; have longer duration; and frequently occur without precipitants. Second, the worries associated with generalized anxiety disorder are excessive and typically interfere significantly with psychosocial functioning, whereas the worries of everyday life are not excessive and are perceived as more manageable and may be put off when more pressing matters arise. The greater the range of life circumstances about which a person worries (e.g., finances, children's safety, job performance), the more likely his or her symptoms are to meet criteria for generalized anxiety disorder. Third, everyday worries are much less likely to be accompanied by physical symptoms (e.g., restlessness or feeling keyed up or on edge). Individuals with generalized anxiety disorder report subjective distress due to constant worry and related impairment in social, occupational, or other important areas of functioning.

21—Generalized Anxiety Disorder / Diagnostic Features (pp. 222–223)

22. A 26-year-old man is brought to the emergency department suffering from a sudden, severe surge of panic. He has no history of panic disorder, but he reports taking several doses of an over-the-counter cold medication earlier that day. Which of the following clinical features, if present in this case, would help to confirm a diagnosis of substance/medication-induced anxiety disorder?

    A. Symptoms that are mild and do not impair functioning.
    B. Symptoms that persist for a long time after substance/medication use.
    C. Symptoms that are in excess of what would be expected for the substance/medication.
    D. Presence of a delirium or gross confusion.
    E. Lack of any history of anxiety disorder or panic symptoms.

    Correct Answer: E. Lack of any history of anxiety disorder or panic symptoms.

    Explanation: Many substances can potentially cause anxiety symptoms, and it can sometimes be difficult to determine whether medication use is etiologically related to the onset of anxiety symptoms. Evidence to support the presence of a substance/medication-induced anxiety disorder includes temporal associations and symptoms that are consistent with the medication and dose. By definition, a substance/medication-induced anxiety disorder must cause significant distress or impairment in functioning, and it cannot occur exclusively during the course of a delirium.

    22—Substance/Medication-Induced Anxiety Disorder / diagnostic criteria; Diagnostic Features (pp. 226–228)

23. In which of the following circumstances would a diagnosis of substance/medication-induced anxiety disorder be appropriate for an individual who stopped taking benzodiazepines the previous day?

    A. Significant anxiety symptoms are present.
    B. Anxiety is present that is clearly related to the withdrawal state.
    C. Anxiety is present that is sufficiently severe to warrant independent clinical attention.
    D. Anxiety is present only during bouts of delirium.
    E. Never: the diagnosis of substance withdrawal would supersede the anxiety disorder diagnosis.

    Correct Answer: C. Anxiety is present that is sufficiently severe to warrant independent clinical attention.

    Explanation: Anxiety symptoms commonly occur in substance intoxication and substance withdrawal. The diagnosis of the substance-specific intoxication or substance-specific withdrawal will usually suffice to categorize the symptom presentation. A diagnosis of substance/medication-induced anxiety disorder should be made in addition to substance intoxication or substance withdrawal only when the panic or anxiety symptoms are predominant in the clinical picture and are sufficiently severe to warrant independent clinical attention.

23—Substance/Medication-Induced Anxiety Disorder / Differential Diagnosis (pp. 229–230)

24. A 60-year-old man has just been diagnosed with congestive heart failure. He is intensely anxious and reports feeling as if he cannot breathe, which causes him to panic. Which of the following features, if present in this case, would tend to support a diagnosis of anxiety disorder due to another medical condition rather than adjustment disorder with anxiety?

    A. The patient says that he is relieved to know his diagnosis.
    B. The patient has no anxiety-associated physical symptoms.
    C. The patient is focused on the reasons he has a cardiac disorder.
    D. The patient is delirious.
    E. The patient is extremely concerned that he will not be able to return to work.

Correct Answer: A. The patient says that he is relieved to know his diagnosis.

Explanation: The essential feature of anxiety disorder due to another medical condition is clinically significant anxiety that is judged to be best explained as a physiological effect of another medical condition. Symptoms can include prominent anxiety symptoms or panic attacks (Criterion A). The judgment that the symptoms are best explained by the associated physical condition must be based on evidence from the history, physical examination, or laboratory findings. In individuals who have serious medical illness and comorbid anxiety symptoms, anxiety disorder due to another medical condition is a potential cause. Anxiety disorder due to another medical condition is more likely to have a physical component of the anxiety than are the adjustment disorders. Anxiety disorder due to another medical condition should be distinguished from adjustment disorders, with anxiety, or with anxiety and depressed mood. Adjustment disorder is warranted when individuals experience a maladaptive response to the stress of having another medical condition. The reaction to stress usually concerns the meaning or consequences of the stress, as compared with the experience of anxiety or mood symptoms that occur as a physiological consequence of the other medical condition. In adjustment disorder, the anxiety symptoms are typically related to coping with the stress of having a general medical condition, whereas in anxiety disorder due to another medical condition, individuals are more likely to have prominent physical symptoms and to be focused on issues other than the stress of the illness itself.

24—Anxiety Disorder Due to Another Medical Condition / Diagnostic Features; Differential Diagnosis (pp. 230–232)